Ursula Markham is a practising hypnotherapist and author of several bestselling books on self-help. In addition to running her own successful clinic, she gives lectures and conducts workshops and seminars in the UK and abroad. She has appeared frequently on radio and television and is Principal of the Hypnothink Foundation, which is responsible for the training of hypnotherapists and counsellors to professional levels.

THE ELEMENT GUIDE SERIES

The Element Guide series addresses important
psychological and emotional issues in a clear,
authoritative and straightforward manner. The
series is designed for all people who deal with these
issues as everyday challenges. Each book explores
the background, possible causes and symptoms
where appropriate, and presents a comprehensive
approach to coping with the situation. Each book
also includes advice on self-help, as well as where –
and when – to turn for qualified help. The books are
objective and accessible, and lead the reader to a
point where they can make informed decisions
about where to go next.

Titles in The Element Guide series:

• THE ELEMENT GUIDE •

MISCARRIAGE

Your Questions Answered

Ursula Markham

ELEMENT

Shaftesbury, Dorset • Boston, Massachusetts
Melbourne, Victoria

First published in Great Britain in 1998 by
Element Books Limited
Shaftesbury, Dorset SP7 8BP

Published in the USA in 1998 by
Element Books, Inc.
160 North Washington Street
Boston, MA 02114

Published in Australia in 1998 by
Element Books and distributed by
Penguin Australia Limited
487 Maroondah Highway
Ringwood, Victoria 3134

Cover illustration by Moira Wills
Cover design by Bridgewater Book Company
Design by Roger Lightfoot
Typeset by WestKey Limited, Falmouth, Cornwall
Printed and bound in Great Britain by
Biddles Ltd, Guildford & Kings Lynn

British Library Cataloguing in Publication
data available

Library of Congress Cataloging in Publication
data available

ISBN 1-86204-297-7

Note from the Publisher
Any information given in any book in *The Element Guide* series is not
intended to be taken as a replacement for medical advice. Any person
with a condition requiring medical attention should consult a qualified
medical practitioner or suitable therapist.

Contents

To Philip and David
With all my love

'On a cloud I saw a child'

WILLIAM BLAKE, *Songs of Innocence*

Introduction

'The loneliest experience I have ever known.' This was how one young woman described her feelings about her recent miscarriage. Even though she had been surrounded by the love and support of her husband, family and friends, she felt that none of them could truly understand what she had been through. And that woman could be considered one of the more fortunate ones; there are many who have to suffer the distress of a miscarriage without the support of a partner or close family member.

Some years ago I was asked to give a talk to the local branch of the Miscarriage Association and, in my role as hypnotherapist and counsellor, to offer any help and advice I could. The talk was intended to be a 'one-off', but I was so moved by the stories of some of these women that I went on to work with many of them on a more long-term basis. To this day I continue to work with those who have joined the group more recently – and it is from that work that this book arises.

As part of my ongoing research I have interviewed many women who have experienced one or more miscarriages, not only those with whom I have worked personally. All the case histories in this book are true – only the names have been changed.

In the book I hope in some way to help deal with the emotions surrounding miscarriage – those of the bereaved mother and of others around her. To help her understand why she feels as she does and to minimize the fears which naturally arise when it comes to future pregnancies.

If you have suffered a miscarriage, or if you know someone who has, this book is for you with my love.

CHAPTER 1

The Loss

'Why me?' The question asked by almost every woman who miscarries. 'What did I do wrong?'

It is really important to realize that a miscarriage is very unlikely to have been caused by anything you did or omitted to do. There are, of course, certain instances where a medical cause can be pinpointed. Some miscarriages, for example, result from the fact that a woman has what is known as an incomplete cervix. This means that the neck of the womb is not strong enough to retain the weight of the developing baby. It opens too soon and a miscarriage results. However, as many as one in four pregnancies can end in miscarriage and, in a substantial number of these cases, no one is able to point to a specific cause.

There are also, of course, basic health rules which it is advisable to follow during pregnancy – cutting out smoking and alcohol, watching your diet, taking rest, etc. – but there are cases of women who have flouted all these rules and gone on to have successful pregnancies while others, who have done everything advised, have not.

A miscarriage can occur in so many different ways. For one woman there will be a short period of discomfort or pain followed almost immediately by what is obviously the loss of her unborn child. Another may experience spotting or light bleeding – even this may start and stop from time to time – and, since many women experience some bleeding during what turns out to be a perfectly successful pregnancy, she may not even realize what is happening to her. Some will have pain in the stomach or the lower part of the back while others will feel no real discomfort at all. Sometimes the feeling is more of an intuitive one – as one woman told me, 'I couldn't put words to what I was feeling; I just knew that something was wrong.'

Yet others may experience a very early miscarriage which might just seem like a late and heavy period. Such women may not even be aware that they had been preg-nant until it shows up at some later examination or until they consider the matter themselves in retrospect and realize what must have happened.

A miscarriage can occur any time up to the end of the twenty-fourth week of pregnancy, after which time it is technically a stillbirth. One of the things many women find difficult to cope with is the fact that, after any initial physical check-up and treatment such as a dilation and curettage, should this prove necessary, there is very little in the way of follow-up assistance available – and in some places none at all. As Diane told me:

> I lost my first baby in the twelfth week of my pregnancy. It took me completely by surprise as I had felt perfectly well when I went to bed but woke in the morning in considerable pain to find that I was bleeding heavily. My husband called the doctor but, by the time he arrived, it was all over.
>
> I had a physical examination which showed that I'd had what they call a 'complete miscarriage' when all the tissue in the uterus has come away and so I didn't even need a dilation and curettage. The doctor was quite kind but told me there was no follow-up treatment available as it was probably 'just one of those things' and that I was quite likely to go on to have a successful pregnancy the next time.
>
> And that was it. No one talked to us, answered our ques-tions, reassured us or gave us any help at all. We were just left in a devastated state to get on with life as though nothing had happened. It didn't help to be told that I couldn't have any tests done or treatment given until I'd had three or more miscarriages.

As it happens, I went on to have two beautiful, healthy daughters in the next four years, but nothing will let me forget the utter desolation I felt when it seemed as though I had been abandoned. If it hadn't been for our local Miscarriage Association group, I don't know what I would have done.

If you feel isolated in this way, do make an appointment to see either your doctor or the health visitor and put to him or her any questions you might have. Even if no one can give you a definite cause for your miscarriage, at least they can explain the possibilities and offer you some reassurance about the future.

Sally's miscarriage was quite different. Because she had shown what could have been threatening symptoms, she was taken into hospital but, despite the care she received there, she lost the baby.

Although, unlike Diana, Sally had realized that she might be about to miscarry, she was naturally deeply distressed. What made things even worse, however, was that she heard the doctor telling the nurse that she had suffered a 'spontaneous abortion'.

While this is the correct medical term for a miscarriage, the word 'abortion' has a completely different meaning in the minds of most people. In many instances now the phrase is avoided where possible as medical staff are sensitive enough to realize the pain it can cause. But, should you hear it said about you or someone you care for, please realize that it is just a medical term and does not imply that anything deliberate has been done to terminate the pregnancy.

Perhaps one of the hardest things for a woman to accept is that, in the case of a miscarriage, she has no control over the situation or over what is happening within her body. One young woman told me that she felt as if the process had taken her over and she was just some sort of machine which was breaking down and there was absolutely nothing she could do about it.

While you may reach a stage where you may not be able to control what is happening to you when the miscarriage is actually taking place, you certainly have the ability to take control afterwards – and it is important that you do. Later in this book we are going to look at the various ways in which you can take control, both of the current sad situation and how you cope with it, and of your physical and emotional state as you contemplate a future pregnancy.

For now, it is extremely important to understand that you have suffered a bereavement. It doesn't matter whether you were in your fourth or fifth month of pregnancy or whether you only found out about your pregnancy a week before. You have lost your child and you should be allowed – and even encouraged – to go through the bereavement process if you are to be able to accept the situation and get on with your life.

There are six main stages of bereavement which we all experience whether we have just lost our 90-year-old grandmother or our unborn child. These are denial, grief, anger, guilt, fear and resentment. Unless you realize that it is normal to experience all these emotions, you may think that there is something wrong with you for doing so.

DENIAL

The denial phase of bereavement may last for a very short or a long period of time. It is a common reaction to the shock of loss where the bereaved person acts as if nothing of great importance has happened and appears to get back to everyday life very quickly. There may be no tears, no verbal expression of how she is feeling, no talk of what might have been. It may seem as though a mother who acts this way after having miscarried is coping exceedingly well, but it is necessary for the sadness to manifest itself. Knowing this, a caring counsellor will gently steer the woman towards expressing her feelings, allowing her to cry or demonstrate any of the other signs of grief which seem appropriate at the time.

This is not as hard-hearted as it might seem. That grief is going to hit home one day and, until it does, the healing process cannot begin.

Margaret was just over three months into her pregnancy when she miscarried. She had only known that she was pregnant for about two weeks before the loss occurred and, apart from her partner and her parents, no one else had known of her condition so she did not have to cope with the words and actions of other people.

Having spent one night in hospital after the miscarriage, Margaret was determined to carry on with her life just as if nothing had happened. She refused to talk about the miscarriage, even to her partner, but rationalized the situation by using all the clichés – it was 'just one of those things'; 'it happens to lots of women'; 'there was probably something wrong with the baby anyway, so it was all for the best'.

She went back to work; she socialized just as she had always done; she worked in her garden. For about four weeks everything seemed just as it had been before. Then, one morning, she awoke to find tears streaming down her face and experiencing a sense of panic which was so great that she did not even think she would be able to get out of bed. She told me:

At first I didn't even connect these feelings with the loss of the baby a month before. After all, I'd seemed to get back to normal so quickly that I really I believed I was 'over it'. Hugh, my partner, didn't make the connection either but he was worried about me and insisted on calling my doctor and making an appointment.

My doctor explained to me that this was a common delayed reaction to the miscarriage and suggested that I go home, take some time off and pamper myself a little until I felt better.

In one way this was helpful as I found I was really tired and, not going to work, I was able to sleep as and when I wanted. But I just could not stop crying – even though it didn't always feel that I was crying about the baby. The thing which frightened me most – and which made me decide to seek counselling – was that I started to make excuses so that I wouldn't have to go out and meet other people. I also felt that

I must be some sort of monster because I hadn't cried for my lost baby since the miscarriage happened – and surely anyone with an ounce of feeling would have done so. I began to think that I didn't deserve to be a mother.

During our sessions together Margaret came to realize that she was not a monster, nor someone who did not deserve to have children, but that everyone reacts differently and on a different timescale to a loss such as she had suffered. She was punishing herself for what she saw as her lack of feeling and this punishment took the form of loss of self-esteem which caused her to be frightened of coming into contact with other people (in case they realized what a 'terrible' person she was).

You may have heard people who have suffered terrible physical injury say that, despite broken bones or damaged organs, they did not feel great pain at the time it happened. Shock had temporarily numbed the pain. Much the same thing had happened in the case of Margaret and women like her; it is as though the pain of their loss is so great that the mind is unable to cope with it immediately and postpones the onset of emotion. But, just as the physical pain eventually returns to the injured person, there comes a time when the mind is faced with the reality of what has happened and all those suppressed emotions come to the fore.

GRIEF

Grief is a healthy reaction to any loss – and probably the one you would be most likely to expect to experience. But, even then, not everyone shows it in the same way.

Most women who have suffered a miscarriage will find it easy to shed tears for the lost baby and for themselves too because, after all, that baby was still a physical part of you. For those who find it difficult to cry or to demonstrate emotion, it is important to find some way of expressing what you feel. You may want to talk about it – whether to someone close to you or to someone who is more detached such as a health visitor or a counsellor. You may even want to write about it.

One of my patients who had always had difficulty with outward demonstration of emotion by herself or others was aware of the pent-up grief within her but did not know how to release it. Her husband was even less emotionally demonstrative than she was and no one else had known of the pregnancy.

I suggested to this woman that she should write a letter to the baby, saying whatever came into her head. She knew that she did not have to show this letter to anyone, but brought it with her the next time she came to see me and asked me to read it.

It was one of the most moving letters I have ever read. It started off quite formally – almost intellectually – as she wrote about the practical things which had happened and her curiosity about how the baby would have turned out had it lived. By the end of the first page, however, there was a marked difference in both the style and content of that letter. She wrote of the love she would have given her child and how she would have cherished him or her (the sex was not known).

At the end of the letter was a short poem telling the lost baby that she (the mother) would go on feeling love for it for the rest of her life, even though they might not meet again until whatever came after this life.

Without realizing that she was doing so, this woman had worked through one of the very important stages of grief and had acknowledged the fact that death does not have to mean the end of love. If we lose a loved parent, friend or partner, we don't immediately stop feeling love for them. We may learn to cope with the loss but the love continues. And, if you believe that there is anything to come after this life, there is absolutely no reason why anyone should cease loving you just because they have died.

ANGER

It often surprises people that anger should be associated with the emotions after a bereavement. It is easy to understand how those who have lost someone because of an accident, a mistake or even a deliberate action on the part of another person can be angry. But why should that particular emotion be connected to an event which, sad though it was, happened spontaneously?

But, although we do not always realize it, anger is a perfectly natural part of the grieving process and deserves to be acknowledged as such. So, if you find yourself experiencing deep anger – whether quietly bitter or loudly vehement – don't worry; there is nothing wrong with you. In fact, although it is best to try not to damage anyone else with your anger, it would be harmful to suppress it completely. It will pass soon enough if acknowledged.

Sometimes the anger felt will appear to have a logical basis. You might feel anger at a doctor, nurse or midwife for failing to anticipate that you might miscarry; or perhaps you are angry at a friend or relative who expects you to be your old self long before you are ready to do so.

At other times the anger is not so logical. You could feel angry when you see families going out together or even angry because the birds are singing. One woman told me how, immediately after her miscarriage, she experienced anger akin to hatred when she saw little children hand in hand with their mother or father. (Strangely it was never the sight of a baby which inflamed her but that of a toddler being cared for by a parent.) When telling me about her emotional state, this young woman confessed that the strength of her anger frightened her. She would never have expressed her anger towards these children and would certainly never have harmed anyone – indeed, she hoped desperately that she hid her feelings well enough at the time so that no one realized they existed. But the fact that she could have them in the first place worried her, and it was only when she realized that they were normal and that they would pass of their own accord that she was able to accept their existence.

GUILT

Feelings of guilt typically follow any bereavement but they are perhaps even more to be found in those who have just experienced miscarriage.

There can't be a woman who has lost a child during pregnancy who hasn't wondered whether perhaps the whole thing was her fault. Suppose she had been more careful about what she ate and drank; if only she had never had those cigarettes; did it all begin when she drove her car too fast on that bumpy road?

In those cases where no reason can be found for the occurrence of the miscarriage, it is all too easy for the woman to blame herself. But – medical conditions apart – it is highly unlikely that, if the pregnancy was progressing satisfactorily in all other respects, any of the things mentioned above would have caused it to end. A poor diet or too much alcohol or smoking during pregnancy may well have a noticeable effect on the baby when it is born – in that it may be smaller and less healthy than it would otherwise have been – but they are very unlikely to have caused the miscarriage of that baby.

It is common, too, for women who have had deliberate terminations of earlier pregnancies to feel that this may be a contributing cause of a later miscarriage. Even when internal examinations prove that no harm has been done and that there are no abnormalities as a result of the abortion, guilt is likely to rear its head.

Angela had become pregnant when she was just 15 years old and still at school. Her parents were very supportive but felt – rightly or wrongly – that to have a child now (whether she kept it or gave it up for adoption) would not be in Angela's best interests. They suggested that she have an abortion as soon as possible. Angela herself was so confused that she did not know what to think – she simply wanted the whole situation to go away. So she went along with her parents' views and an abortion was carried out at a sleek and expensive private clinic. Afterwards Angela was examined and found to have no physical ill effects, although she was naturally distressed at first.

In her mid-twenties Angela married Fraser and about six months later she was pregnant with their first child. All went well until the fourth month of that pregnancy when sadly Angela suffered a miscarriage. Because no one could give her a reason why this should have happened, Angela convinced herself that it must all be her fault and that she was being 'punished' for having had an abortion all those years ago. Perhaps she did not deserve to have a baby; perhaps this was God's way of punishing her; perhaps she would never have a baby of her own.

None of this was true, of course. Whether or not you agree with the concept of abortion, all that had happened when Angela was very young and under the influence of parents who did what they thought best for her. And, if you accept the existence of God (or Spirit, or whatever other name you care to use), surely a force of good which is so wise would never be petty enough to act on a tit-for-tat basis.

Angela needed to understand that, because guilt is a normal part of the grieving process and she was going to experience it anyway, her mind had latched on to that earlier stage in her life as a focal point. It was probable that there had always been an underlying sense of guilt there and her current tragedy had simply served to enhance it. In Angela's case it was necessary not only to deal with her feelings after her recent miscarriage but also to go into her feelings about the earlier abortion, using a combination of hypnotherapy and counselling to work through those feelings which she had been suppressing for so long.

Barbara's sense of guilt after her miscarriage also led her to feel that she was being punished, but for a different reason.

She and her husband Don were both professional people who were doing well in their respective careers. If they thought about having children at all, it would not be for several years as they were both enjoying living the 'high life' while they were young.

Then suddenly, despite taking what they considered to be sufficient precaution, Barbara found that she was pregnant. She was not happy. She was just about to take another step up the ladder in her career, she and Don had a busy social life, they lived in a luxurious apartment in the centre of town . . . there was nowhere in this scenario for disturbed nights, nappies and teething.

The couple discussed the possibility of an abortion but each felt that, although they had not wanted the pregnancy, they did not feel able to terminate it coldly and deliberately. Eventually they decided that they would move to a house on the outskirts of town and that, once the baby was born, they would employ a full-time nanny so that Barbara could continue with her career. But how she wished that she had never become pregnant.

As the weeks passed, however, Barbara found that she was quite enjoying the thought of being a mother. She became quite emotional when she felt those first tiny, fluttering movements within her. She began to think about names, prams and nurseries.

Then it happened. One day she was pregnant, feeling fit and well and enjoying life, and the next she was lying in a hospital bed having suffered a miscarriage. No warning and no explanation. 'Just one of those things,' they told her.

But, like Angela, Barbara didn't think it was just one of those things. The guilt she naturally experienced as part of her bereavement convinced her that it was all her fault – that the baby knew it was unwanted and chose not to come to unloving parents. If only she'd never said that she wished she were not pregnant; she would give anything now to feel her child moving within her.

Once again, this was a case of normal emotions looking for something to latch on to. In Barbara's case there was a ready-made hook – she had never wanted to be pregnant in the first place. But, just as in Angela's case, Barbara had to see that that thought in itself could not have caused the miscarriage. If such wishes were strong enough to do so, then no unwanted pregnancies would ever reach full term and we all know that this is not the case.

FEAR

We have looked at the four emotions which commonly accompany any form of bereavement, but there is a fifth one which is common to almost every woman who experiences a miscarriage: fear. Fear that she may never become pregnant again; fear that she will not be able to carry a baby to full term; fear that her husband or partner will not want to stay with her if she is unable to have children.

Obviously there are some miscarriages which are caused by some physical condition which may be temporary and able to respond to treatment or which may be permanent. In either of those cases help should be sought from the relevant professionals – whether doctors, consultant obstetricians, adoption agencies, etc.

Even in those cases when there is no physical cause, the fear exists just the same. There are various points to bear in mind:

- You shouldn't feel foolish for experiencing this fear – it is quite natural and, indeed, it would be surprising if you did not feel it.
- Fear itself is one of the great causes of stress and tension in any person and it is an acknowledged fact that a woman who is suffering from deep stress is far less likely to become pregnant. So, while accepting and acknowledging the existence of the fear, try to find some method of relaxing – whether by practising yoga or having treatment such as hypnotherapy or aromatherapy.

• A husband or partner who loves you is not going to leave you even if you were not able to have children. (If he did, he would not be worth having in the first place and certainly would not have made a good father.) But it is important to remember that he may be suffering too. I know the grief can never be quite the same as it is for the woman because the baby has never been a physical part of him. And, particularly when they are trying hard to be strong for the sake of their wives, men often find it difficult to put their feelings into words.

Talk together; cry together if necessary; go through all the healing processes together – and your relationship will be enhanced rather than harmed by the tragedy you have suffered.

RESENTMENT

Resentment is also something quite often experienced by those who have suffered a miscarriage. Sometimes these feelings are justified and sometimes they are not. It is quite common to feel that the doctor should have been aware that something was wrong, that a physical examination should have shown that all was not well or that the mother herself should have realized that things were not right.

Although these feelings are understandable, it has been shown that, in those cases where a reason can be found for the miscarriage, about 50 per cent of them take place because of some defect or abnormality in the foetus. So early knowledge would have made no difference to the situation or the outcome. In some cases there is not even a foetus at all but simply placenta and membranes – known as a 'blighted ovum'.

There are cases, however, where that feeling of resentment may well be justified. Some doctors and some hospitals lack the sensitivity which should be paramount when dealing with a woman who is in the process of losing her unborn baby. This is by no means an indictment of all doctors, nurses or hospitals as some go out of their way to demonstrate their compassionate understanding of the situation. And everyone realizes that the medical professions are under great stress due to pressure of work and financial restraints. Nonetheless, it takes little extra time and thought to deal sensitively with a woman suffering a miscarriage.

CHAPTER 2

The Early Miscarriage

Years ago it was not possible to have tests to be sure you were pregnant until you had missed two, or even three, periods. Only then could you go to your doctor for a check-up – and, of course, by that time you often had other symptoms, such as morning sickness or tender breasts, to give you a pretty good idea.

Now, however, things have become much more sophisticated. Couples are much more aware of optimum ovulation times, home pregnancy testing kits are available to anyone, so it is possible to know you are pregnant almost from the very beginning.

This can be wonderful if the pregnancy is wanted and if all goes well. But it also means that some women who experience a very early miscarriage are all too aware of the fact – whereas in the past some of them would merely have thought they were having a late and heavy period.

Early miscarriage refers to one which takes place any time from conception until about the sixteenth week.

It is far more common than most people realize for a miscarriage to take place within this time, often for no known reason. The good news, however, is that the majority of women who suffer an early miscarriage, particularly during their first pregnancy, go on to have perfectly normal pregnancies afterwards.

When Sandra and Ray got married, they decided that they would like children as soon as possible. So they were both delighted when, about six months later, a home pregnancy testing kit showed that Sandra was pregnant. When she telephoned her doctor to make an appointment for an examination and test, the doctor told her to wait until the twelfth week before coming in.

Sandra did not experience any particular symptoms in those first few weeks – no morning sickness, no tenderness in the breasts. Indeed, had it not been for the test she had done using the kit, she would not even have realized she was pregnant.

In her eighth week– at what would have been the time of her second missed period – Sandra noticed that she had lost a few spots of blood but nothing dramatic. She telephoned the doctor and was told that this was not unusual. In fact she knew this for herself as her older sister, Jan, had experienced the same thing during both her pregnancies but had gone on to give birth to a healthy son on each occasion.

A week later, however, the spotting turned to heavy bleeding accompanied by stomach cramps and discomfort rather than by severe pain. The doctor was called and Sandra was taken into hospital but nothing could be done and she had a miscarriage.

As she told me later, if Sandra had not used the testing kit, she would probably not have realized that she was pregnant in the first place and, because her periods were sometimes late and were often accompanied by stomach cramps, she would just have assumed that this was what had happened in this case.

This doesn't mean that home testing is a bad thing or that it is not a good idea to know you are pregnant as soon as possible. What it does mean, however, is that many more women are aware of having had an early miscarriage than would formerly have been the case.

One of the deepest regrets of women who suffer a very early miscarriage is that they feel they have nothing to mourn. It is hard to link the loss of blood and tissue with the concept of a baby and it is not unusual for such women to feel almost cheated.

'Just look on it as a heavy period' was the 'comfort' offered to one woman. 'Oh well, you can always try again,' another was told. But these women had lost their babies and to them this was a bereavement and a cause for grief, no matter how short the pregnancy had been.

Bleeding of any sort can be one of the indications of an impending miscarriage – but, as already said, it is not uncommon and can also be something which happens during what turns out to be a normal and successful pregnancy. But, if you experience bleeding – even light spotting – and you are concerned, go to bed and call your doctor, if only to have your mind put at rest.

Bleeding during pregnancy often stops when the woman lies down, only to begin again when she gets up. This can cause a dreadful seesaw of emotions because at one moment you feel as though everything is going to be all right and, at the next, all those anxieties return.

If this is your situation, it is possible to request an ultrasound scan which will show whether the baby is developing at the normal rate. Remember, however, that a heartbeat may be extremely difficult to detect at this very early stage – even when all is well – so lack of that sound is not necessarily a cause for concern unless there are other indications of problems.

One of the problems in such cases is that you may have to wait several days for a scan and this prolongs the period of uncertainty, leaving you with your emotions riding on the rollercoaster of hope and despair. Hard as it may be, if you find yourself caught in such a waiting period, try to remain as calm and relaxed as possible as stress and tension can be great enemies at such a time.

When a woman has requested an early scan because she has some apprehension about the progress of her pregnancy and that scan proves that her fears were soundly based, it does not make the fact of the miscarriage easier to bear, but it does avoid the shock element which can occur at the time of the first routine scan.

Rachel was delighted to find that she was pregnant. She felt extremely well during those first weeks – not even a hint of morning sickness.

When the time came for her first routine scan, she went along quite happily, looking forward to the new experience which would show her how her baby was developing. Her first indication that anything might be wrong was when everyone went very quiet and no one spoke to her. The operator left the room and she could see him through a window talking rapidly to the auxiliary in the next room. Then he returned and said that a doctor would be along to speak to her in a few moments.

Had it not been for the awkwardness in his manner, Rachel might not have felt that anything was wrong. This was her first scan and she was not quite sure what was normal procedure.

Several minutes later a doctor came into the room and watched the screen as she was scanned again. Then he dropped the bombshell. He told Rachel that the scan showed clearly that the foetus had failed to develop naturally and that, although she had shown no outwards signs of it, she had in fact suffered a miscarriage. All that remained now was for her to have a complete evacuation of the retained products of conception (often known as an ERPC). Many people still call this process a dilation and curettage – or even a 'scrape' – but, strictly speaking, a dilation and curettage is what takes place after a pregnancy.

When I met Rachel some weeks after her scan she was physically perfectly well but emotionally she was still in a very shaky state. The shock of realizing that she was no longer pregnant was very difficult for her to come to terms with. In addition to the distress she naturally felt was the feeling that her body had betrayed her and she could no longer trust it.

'I felt so well,' she told me. 'I didn't have the faintest idea that anything could be wrong. I don't think I'll ever be able to trust my feelings about myself again. I'll never know whether I'm suffering from some terrible illness if my body keeps secrets from me like that.'

In that case Rachel felt resentful that her body had 'let her down' by giving no indication that anything was going wrong. As it happens, she was assured that, even had she known that there was a problem at an earlier stage, there would have been absolutely nothing that could have been done about it. But this did not relieve her feelings and now she had an extra emotional dimension to add to the sense of loss and sorrow which naturally accompany any miscarriage.

After Caroline lost the child she was expecting during the twelfth week of her pregnancy, it was necessary for her to spend a few days in hospital. Perhaps the hospital in question was overcrowded, or perhaps no one even paused to consider Caroline's feelings. For whatever reason, she was put in a ward with five other women, two of whom required bed rest during the last few days of their pregnancy and three of whom had just given birth to perfectly healthy babies.

Everywhere she looked in that ward Caroline saw signs of happy and successful pregnancies and this only served to heighten her already fragile emotions at the loss of her own unborn child. The other five women were so engrossed in their talk of feeding, nappies and names that, after initially commiserating with Caroline on her loss, they tended to leave her out of any conversations. They did not mean to be unkind but, for one thing, they probably did not know quite what to say to her and, for another, their minds were full of this wonderful event which had just taken place, or was just about to take place, in their own lives.

Caroline did not mind that they didn't include her in their chatter – after all, how could she talk enthusiastically about new babies and their needs – but she did resent the fact that, wherever she turned, there was a happy mother and a healthy baby before her eyes. She asked to be moved from that particular ward but was told there was nowhere else for her to go. It was only when she became quite hysterical during an evening visit that her husband created a fuss and *insisted* that something be done. Caroline was then put in a small side ward by herself and, though naturally still unhappy about her own condition, at least she did not have to spend all day being reminded about what she might have had.

In this case Caroline and her husband believed that their feelings of resentment were justified. Not only were the staff concerned insensitive enough to put her in that ward in the first place, but they were not compassionate enough to respond to her pleas for a change until she reached such a hysterical state that her health was threatened.

How a woman is told that she has miscarried – or that she is likely to do so – is very important and greatly affects her wellbeing in the immediate future after the event. Of course she is going to be upset and no amount of kind words and phrases can change that; but there is a great deal of difference between having the news broken to you by a caring and sympathetic individual – whether doctor, nurse or scan operator – and hearing the sad reality as a cold, stark fact.

Some medical practitioners are wonderful when it comes to dealing with the emotions of their patients, but this is due more to their innate sensitivity and compassion than to any training they may have had. At the time of writing there is often no official training given in how to break this sort of news to a patient and, sad as it is to report, the experiences related to me by women I have treated after a miscarriage seem to indicate that there are still all too many professionals who see only the medical condition and not the human being involved.

A miscarriage – particularly one which takes place in the early weeks of pregnancy – can occur in many different ways. Sometimes it is a sudden happening, sometimes there may be minor symptoms which drag on over several days and sometimes the mother does not even realize what has happened until she is told after a scan or examination.

Elaine was one of those whose miscarriage during the early weeks of her pregnancy seemed to go on for days with symptoms which grew progressively more severe. She suffered a fair amount of pain and there was also a good deal of blood loss. 'I didn't realize it could drag on so,' she told me, 'or that it could be so messy – there was such a lot of blood.'

When I first saw Elaine about four weeks after her miscarriage, the memory and the pictures were still to the forefront of her mind. She was frightened that she would never be able to get rid of them. By means of hypnotherapy it was possible to allow these thoughts and images to fade so that, although she would never forget what had happened, they no longer loomed so large or affected her so greatly. And, although at that time she stated adamantly that she had given up all thoughts of having children because she was never going to risk going through all that again, Elaine is now the proud mother of two boys and a girl.

Blood is something which frightens many women, particularly when it seems excessive, as it can when experiencing a miscarriage. Even those who experience slight spotting during what turns out to be a normal and successful pregnancy, are apprehensive in case the flow increases and causes them – or others – to become embarrassed. In fact, if you speak to women who have suffered a miscarriage, the amount of blood is something which seems to stick in their minds long after memories of other physical symptoms have begun to recede. Also, it is quite normal for there to be bleeding after a miscarriage and it may well continue until the first proper period after the miscarriage. However, it is important to inform your doctor at once if you are in pain, if the blood you lose is clotted, or if you feel feverish.

Because of the amount of blood, I have known women who contemplated avoiding the ERPC, but it is really important for this procedure to be carried out, as it will ensure that all is well and avoid the risk of any infection setting in. Unless you have suffered a complete miscarriage –

which is not common in the early stages of pregnancy –
failure to have an ERPC could seriously affect your chances
of a future successful pregnancy.

Margaret initially refused an ERPC after her miscarriage.
She felt that it was the last straw, that she could not bear to
be 'messed about with' (as she put it) any more. What had
happened already had been beyond her control and she felt
she had lost the ability to be in charge of her own body. It
was only after gentle persuasion from her husband and a
nurse that she agreed to go ahead – something which I am
sure she came to appreciate at a later date.

Any miscarriage is hard to cope with but those which
take place in the early weeks of pregnancy often happen
to women who are expecting their first child. Not only do
they have the sad event itself to deal with but there is usually a fear – often unspoken – that they will never be able
to go on to have children in the future. Happily this is not
the case and the great majority of those who suffer such
an early miscarriage do in fact go on to have successful
pregnancies.

CHAPTER 3

The Late Miscarriage

A late miscarriage (that is one which takes place after the sixteenth week) is far less common than an early one. It is also far more likely that a recognizable cause can be found for a late miscarriage. Perhaps the woman has gone into labour too soon or it could be that the baby has died in the womb. In a small number of instances it could be that there was some external cause, such as a fall or an accident of some sort, which has led to the miscarriage.

Extreme stress is also a factor to consider. Although this is unlikely to be the sole cause of a miscarriage, it can certainly contribute to one if other conditions already exist. This is why it is such a good idea for *all* pregnant women to practise a deep relaxation technique throughout the whole of their pregnancy. (You will find such a technique detailed in the self-help chapter of this book.)

Bridget and her husband John had just spent a lovely day with John's parents. Bridget was 18 weeks pregnant with her first child and had felt extremely well for the whole of that time. She and John (and their respective families) were eagerly anticipating what was to be the first grandchild on each side of the family.

It was dusk as John drove carefully home through the country lanes. There was very little traffic around until suddenly, as if from nowhere, a small red sports car roared up behind them. Although they were approaching a bend in the road, the driver of the sports car decided to overtake – just as another car appeared coming towards them. Trying to avoid a collision, the driver of the sports car pulled in suddenly in front of them, clipping the front of their car as he did so. John did all he could but was unable to prevent their car being forced off the narrow road and into a ditch.

Fortunately, no one was hurt in the accident but the car belonging to John and Bridget suffered quite a bit of damage, including a broken axle, so they had to wait for one of the rescue services to come and take them home. John's concern for Bridget made him extremely angry and he wasted no words in telling the young driver of the sports car just what he thought of him.

Bridget had initially been terrified that the impact and the jolting, combined with the stress of the situation, would do her and her baby some harm, but all seemed to be well and she arrived home some time later having recovered from the shock of the accident.

It was the middle of the night when she became aware that something was very wrong. She experienced terrible stomach cramps and she started to bleed. John lost no time in calling an ambulance and very soon Bridget was being examined in hospital. Sadly they could do nothing and by morning she had miscarried.

There was, of course, an insurance claim to be settled after the accident and, with the driver of the oncoming car as a witness, the blame was laid squarely on the young man with the sports car. But, although the car was repaired and Bridget was awarded a small sum for the pain and distress she had suffered during that night, there was no element of compensation for the loss of her unborn baby's life.

This was something Bridget found very hard to accept and one of the main reasons why she consulted me in the first place. It wasn't that she was after a sum of money – no amount of cash could bring her baby back – but she felt angry that the child she had been carrying seemed not to count at all, as if it had never existed. What she really wanted was some official acknowledgement that a life had been lost and the fact that this was not forthcoming was something she found very difficult to accept.

By the time you reach the sixteenth week of pregnancy, you have had much more time to think about motherhood and generally to get used to the idea of being pregnant. Even in those cases where the pregnancy was not wanted at first, the mother has usually had time to come to terms with the idea now and has probably begun to make plans and think about her baby's future.

A late miscarriage is a far more public event. Depending upon the stage of pregnancy reached, you will either have told other people about it or your increasing size will have made the situation obvious. You may have begun to make definite decisions – names you like, the type of pram you want, what colour to have the nursery . . . In some cases the shopping or the decorating may already have begun.

You will have felt the movement of your child within you; you may have been helped to hear its heartbeat. You will have seen the ultrasound scan and perhaps been given a photograph to take home with you. You may even have learned the baby's sex.

In some cases, because of the position in which the baby is lying, it is not possible to tell whether it is a boy or girl. Where it can be seen, the scan operator will usually ask the parents whether or not they wish to know the sex of their child. Some parents want to know as early as possible while others prefer to wait until the baby is born.

Without exception, every woman I have spoken to who has suffered a miscarriage has found that it helped enormously to know the sex of the baby she has lost. Referring to the infant as 'he' or 'she' instead of 'it' or just 'the baby' made it seem part of the family – someone she could talk about and grieve for. When it is a late miscarriage, it is possible for the doctor, nurse or midwife to identify the sex of the baby even if it had not been ascertained beforehand.

This is not always the case with an early miscarriage, even if an ultrasound scan has taken place.

No one was ever able to tell Claire the sex of her baby. There had been a scan but the baby was lying in such a way that it was impossible to discern the sex. Initially this upset Claire very much – it seemed to make her baby a 'thing' rather than a person. So she followed her intuition and decided that she felt the baby to be a girl. She named her Ruth. Doing this made the grieving process seem much more natural and helped Claire to get through the sad time which follows a miscarriage.

Particularly when expecting a first child, each stage of the pregnancy is a new experience. Even with subsequent children, it is possible for each pregnancy to be different. So it is hard for any woman to be sure whether what she is feeling is a normal part of pregnancy or an indication that something is wrong. Some babies' movements are quite gentle, while others seem to be practising for a place in a football team! Some mothers feel healthier and happier during their pregnancy than at any other time, while others, even if not ill, never seem to be free of aches, pains and twinges. Moods can be affected too, with some women alternating been highs and lows – excitement and anxiety – while others remain calm and serene throughout. All these things – particularly when happening for the first time – are accepted as a normal part of pregnancy, making it easy to miss the early warning signs of a miscarriage.

This does not mean that you should go to the other extreme and worry about every ache or twinge and whether it is a sign of impending doom. But, should anything happen which you have not been led to believe is a common part of pregnancy, it is better to ask for a check-up than to soldier on and see what happens.

Take the breaking of your waters, for example. If this occurs during pregnancy, it should be taken as a sign that all is not well. Naturally, if they break all at once, you will hardly fail to notice what has happened. But it is also possible for it to happen gradually.

From about the twentieth week of her pregnancy Felicity became aware of a slight loss of water on a daily basis. But she felt no pain or discomfort and she did not realize that this was actually the breaking of her waters (she imagined that this would come with a gush – as indeed it usually does) so she did nothing about it, assuming that this was part of what happens during a normal pregnancy.

Then, about a fortnight later, Felicity realized that she was feeling very tired and had little energy. So she made an appointment to see her doctor and was dismayed to find herself being rushed into hospital. Her waters had, in fact, broken and her baby had died in the womb.

No matter how often the medical staff tried to assure her that, even if she had realized what was happening a fortnight earlier, it was unlikely that the miscarriage could have been prevented, Felicity could not forgive herself for what she thought of as her own negligence and she always wondered whether possibly her baby might have lived if she had sought help earlier.

A woman who suffers a late miscarriage may well experience exactly the same feelings – physical and emotional – as one who has given birth to a healthy baby. Because the baby, in most cases, has developed considerably, it will be larger and therefore there will be little difference between the pain and effort involved in miscarriage or in childbirth.

The hormonal disturbance may also be the same so that, as well as having to contend with her distress at losing her baby, the woman who has miscarried can also suffer from post-natal depression. Not everyone experiences post-natal depression after giving birth to a healthy child, but those who do know that the condition can last anything from a day or so to several months. It always passes – either with or without professional assistance. There can be few hypnotherapists who have not helped new mothers to overcome the effects of 'baby blues'. But when that condition is augmented by sadness at the loss of the baby it is even more important for help to be sought.

Teresa had no real problems with her first two pregnancies and her daughters were aged seven and four when she found herself expecting her third child. She and her husband Tom were delighted and, at first, the pregnancy appeared to be as trouble-free as the two earlier ones had been.

Then, at the beginning of the twenty-second week, Teresa knew that something was wrong. She began to experience intermittent pains which felt to her just like the contractions she had known when giving birth to her two daughters.

Because these pains seemed to start and stop at intervals for no apparent reason – it made no difference whether Teresa had been active or resting – she was not sure if they were, in fact, contractions. Perhaps she was imagining it. Should she consult her doctor or not? She knew that all pregnancies were not necessarily the same and, just because she had not had any problems before, did not mean that these pains were an indication that something was wrong. After all, she was several years older than she had been when expecting the girls.

Every time she tried to force herself to think positively about the situation, a little voice would pop into Teresa's mind. But suppose something *is* wrong – how will you feel if you don't seek help? Suppose the baby is born far too early and there is something seriously wrong? Suppose you are actually going to lose the baby? The stress she was experiencing seemed to add strength to those pains.

Teresa went to bed and Tom called their doctor. He took one look at Teresa and immediately sent her to hospital. There the pains subsided and it seemed as though all would be well. But the next day they were back and stronger than ever – and this time there were no periods of respite. That night Teresa lost her baby.

No one ever pretends that childbirth is easy or pain-free. Indeed, many women who have just given birth vow that they will never go through that experience again. But labour pains are soon forgotten when there is the joy – and hard work – of a new-born baby in the family. When there is no new-born baby, however, those pains seem doubly cruel.

Teresa told me that she felt 'cheated'. She had experienced the pains of labour when her daughters were born and had been quite prepared for them this time. But to go through all that and find herself without a baby at the end of it – this seemed so unfair. Because of that, the memory of those contractions and the pain she had felt stayed with her far longer than it might otherwise have done.

Some miscarriages result from the fact that a woman has what is known as an incomplete cervix. This means that the neck of the womb is not strong enough to retain the weight of the developing baby. It opens too soon and a miscarriage results.

Once this condition has been diagnosed, it is quite a simple procedure to insert a cervical stitch and so keep the neck of the womb closed during future pregnancies. But, because a woman is not considered to have a real problem unless she has suffered three miscarriages, the condition is not necessarily diagnosed until that time. It is possible, however, to request an examination to determine whether you are one of those women with an incomplete cervix after your first miscarriage. If you are, preventative action can be taken at an earlier stage than might otherwise be the case and you might be saved future heartache.

For many women – and their partners too – a great deal of fear accompanies an actual or threatened miscarriage. Not only fear of the miscarriage itself but fear of what 'it' will look like. Will it be like a baby or, as one young woman put it, like a 'large blood clot'? How messy will the whole process be and how much of it will they see?

These are perfectly natural fears for anyone facing a situation they have never encountered before. The trouble is that many couples – who are already in a state of distress and anxiety – are scared to ask these questions in case it makes them seem ignorant. This would not be the case and their questions would be answered honestly but staff, who may be coping as kindly and efficiently as possible with what is happening, don't always realize what the couple want to know.

Gill is a nurse on the gynaecological ward of a Gloucestershire hospital and I met her when she came to talk to a meeting of the local group of the Miscarriage Association. She explained that it is very difficult to know how much to say when a woman is going through a miscarriage. Some people take the attitude that they just want to close their eyes and get the whole, horrible situation over and done with. Others really need explanations and reassurance as things progress.

Gill told us about a young girl of seventeen who was in the process of suffering a miscarriage. The girl was terrified and clung on to Gill's hand, saying nothing. 'I didn't know how much she would want me to say,' Gill told me. 'She was in tears and I felt that it wouldn't take much for me to start crying too – she looked so young and vulnerable and she was so frightened. In the end I didn't say anything much. I just tried to be as comforting as possible.'

Hospital staff are in a very difficult position. They may want to be as helpful as possible but have no way of knowing what each individual already knows or what they want to know. There is no point in giving graphic details to someone who cannot cope with them, yet others might feel better if they knew just what to expect. So if you have any questions about the miscarriage – either at the time or later when it is all over – do ask for the information you want.

If it is found that the baby has already died, it may be necessary for labour to be artificially induced. This is a process which can take several hours – sometimes longer than a natural birth – and involves the use of a drip.

Sadly this procedure can be as uncomfortable or as painful as normal labour – and the fear and dismay obviously being experienced by the mother can add to her stress and tension, making it very difficult for her to cooperate with any instructions she may be given.

This was the situation in which Hannah found herself. As she told me, 'They kept telling me to "push" but I didn't want to. My mind knew perfectly well what was happening and that my baby was no longer alive, but part of me just wanted to hold on to him for as long as I possibly could. I knew that, once I did as they asked and let him go, he would be gone for ever. I just needed to hold on to him for that little bit longer. The nurse said that I was just being difficult.'

The way in which the mother is treated at what cannot help but be a difficult and distressing time makes an enormous difference to her perception of events and to her feelings when it is all over. Two women with whom I have worked told me of their very different experiences.

'The hospital staff were absolutely wonderful,' said Gabrielle. 'They treated both me and my baby with the utmost dignity. Immediately after it happened they wrapped her in a clean white towel as a shawl and gave her to me to hold. She looked so tiny and so perfect. Paul, my partner, was with me and he held her too. The staff went away and left us, telling us we could have as long with our daughter as we wanted. We were able to talk together and cry together and to tell our baby girl how much we loved her and were going to miss her. When we felt able to give her up, the nurse carried her away as gently and carefully as if she were alive, leaving Paul with me for as long as we wished.'

Helena's experience was very different indeed. 'Before I really knew what was happening, they rushed away with something wrapped in paper towels. I never saw my baby, never had a chance to hold him. I don't even know for certain what sex the baby was but I couldn't bear thinking of an "it" so I decided to believe that he was a boy. I've even given him a name – I've called him Peter. I just wish I'd had a chance to hold him, even if only for a minute.'

Many women will feel nervous about holding their baby after a miscarriage, not knowing how they will feel and whether they will be able to bear to look at the infant. But

I have worked with many, many women who have suffered miscarriages and I don't know of a single case of a woman who has regretted looking at and holding her child. It makes the baby a real person rather than a medical condition and can prove to be extremely comforting for both the mother and her partner.

Many hospitals are now very good about allowing – and even encouraging – this contact between mother and baby. It is greatly to be hoped that in time every hospital will act in the same way.

Mothers are often sent home almost immediately after a miscarriage, unless there are any physical complications. If an ERPC is needed, a woman may be kept in hospital until the following day. (With a late miscarriage it is not always necessary to have an ERPC as the placenta often comes away naturally.)

As far as the hospital is concerned, there is nothing more to be done. The woman is not ill, she does not need medical attention nor does she belong in a maternity ward. So they send her home. But no one tells her what to expect or what to do. No doctor comes to see her; she is just left to get on with it.

A woman who has just suffered a late miscarriage may still be in pain and is probably still suffering from shock. She will naturally be distressed at her loss and fearful about what the future might hold. Her breasts may be tender and she may find that she begins to produce milk. If this should happen to you, don't be tempted to try to express the milk in the hope that you will get rid of it. All that will happen is that you will stimulate its production. If it doesn't stop naturally in a few days, it is possible to get help from your doctor, either by means of tablets or injections.

Once at home, even if she soon feels physically well again, there are so many difficult things to be done. People who knew about the pregnancy have to be told and this should be done quite soon to save embarrassment on all sides. If a friend telephones for a chat and breezily asks how the pregnancy is progressing, not only will all the distress come to the fore again but the caller is going to feel awkward and uncomfortable and may even be put off calling again – and this is a time when friends can prove invaluable.

The easiest way to cope with this situation is to tell immediate family and ask them to pass the news on to other friends and relatives. It might be too traumatic a piece of news for the grieving parents to relate for themselves.

Another difficulty which arises with a late miscarriage is that the mother may return to a home where she is surrounded by preparations for the baby she has now lost. Perhaps a room has been decorated as a nursery; there may be a brand-new pram in the hall; there are probably baby clothes and toys lovingly placed in preparation for their new owner. If the hospital stay has been minimal, there will have been no time for these to have been removed from immediate sight. Indeed, this may not be the best thing to do in any case. Some women find that they cannot bear to see all these signs of the baby they have lost, while others find great comfort in touching and handling toys, clothes, etc. They serve almost as a memorial to their baby.

Because there is no right or wrong way of handling this situation, it is important initially to go along with what the mother wants. If she cannot bear to enter the nursery at first, she should not be made to do so. But if it brings her comfort to sit in there in those early days, no one should prevent her. Either extreme reaction will pass in time. It is similar to those who have suffered other forms of bereavement, some of whom will clear out wardrobes and cupboards almost immediately, while others need to keep those tangible reminders of the person they have lost for a while longer.

When a woman has suffered a miscarriage she often feels extremely isolated. Other people do not always know how to handle the situation. Should they leave the mother (or the couple) to her (their) grief or should they call and see her? If they do call, what on earth are they going to say?

If you know of someone who has recently miscarried, please just be there. It doesn't matter what you say; it doesn't matter if you don't say anything – there aren't any 'right'; words, after all. But what she will need more than anything is to know that people care and that they are there for her to lean on, talk to or cry on when she needs it.

When Judith first went home after losing her baby in the twenty-second week of her pregnancy, her mother and her husband both took time off work to stay with her and make sure she was not alone. But the time came when they had to go back to their respective jobs and that was when the sense of isolation set in.

As Judy told me,

> No one came to see me and, after the first week or so, people stopped telephoning. Perhaps my friends were embarrassed; most of them already have young children and they might have felt it would make me feel worse whatever they did. Bringing their babies or toddlers with them might serve as too painful a reminder of what I had lost. If they came without them, they probably wouldn't know whether to talk about them and risk upsetting me or not to mention them at all, which would be so obvious that it would press the point home even more dramatically. So they just didn't come.
>
> Eventually I bumped into one couple in the supermarket and they asked me if I was 'feeling better now'. I know they meant well but it made it seem as if I'd had nothing more serious than a bout of flu.

Another poignant moment to be faced is the dawning of the day on which the baby was due to be born. Because, in the case of a late miscarriage, this is likely to be only a few weeks after the loss, it is bound to be a difficult time. It is often helpful to try to look on that day as a memorial to the brief time the baby existed and to mark it in a way which seems appropriate to you.

Of all the women I have worked with and those I have interviewed, the majority say that the date only has real significance in the year of the miscarriage itself. As one of my patients put it: 'When you think about it from a greater distance, a life is a life and a death is a death. Dates are numbers on a calendar and don't really mean anything at all.'

After losing a baby you might want to arrange a proper burial service or cremation. In the UK, any baby born alive before 24 weeks and all babies born after 24 weeks must be buried or cremated by law. Before that time the decision is yours.

Some hospitals will help with the arrangements for such a ceremony – or you might prefer to arrange it yourself. It is not even necessary for it to be a religious ceremony – this will depend upon your own beliefs. Even though the day may be a sad one, you will probably appreciate the opportunity both to acknowledge the existence of your baby and to have a chance to say a proper goodbye.

CHAPTER 4

In Loving Memory

The use of language is a strange thing. Women who are pregnant place a different emphasis on different words. One woman will think of herself as a 'mother' from the very moment the pregnancy is confirmed; another will simply say that she is 'pregnant' or even 'expecting'. One will talk about her pregnancy almost as though it is just a medical condition while the other will refer to 'my baby' even at a time when it is known that the foetus has not yet developed.

Because of their use of different words or phrases, a miscarriage may have a somewhat different effect on each woman. If the miscarriage is an early one, the emotional effect may be greater on the woman who has thought about the baby from the very beginning.

I am not suggesting here that you would be wiser to think only of 'pregnancy' for as long as possible, keeping all thoughts of the child within you to one side. You will do what comes naturally to you – and that is just as it should be.

There are legal definitions which apply to pregnancy and the time at which the 'foetus' becomes a 'baby', but these really bear no reference to the way people feel. Apart from each woman's instinctive reactions, there are cultural and religious differences in belief. Some people believe that the foetus is a human being with a spirit or a soul from the moment of conception while others do not consider this to be so until the moment of birth.

The difference in use of language (and therefore of the thought behind the language) is not only apparent in relation to the pregnancy but applies if anything should go wrong with that pregnancy. While one woman will say that she has 'had a miscarriage', another will say that she has 'lost the baby'. The former may find it easier to use words which make it appear that she has suffered from a temporary medical condition while the latter feels the need to give status and reality to the child she was carrying.

The stage of pregnancy reached may also have some bearing on how each woman thinks and the words she uses. While many do not think of 'the baby' until they have seen their child on the ultrasound scan or felt it move within them – and while a few don't consider the baby a separate person until the moment of birth – there are others who think and talk of the 'baby' from the moment they miss their first period and have the pregnancy confirmed.

Women who have been planning their pregnancy for some time or who have had difficulty in conceiving are more likely to think in terms of 'the baby' from very early on.

Katy and her husband Jack had been married for four years and for the last two of those years they had been trying for a baby with no result. Finally they went for tests, only to discover that Jack had a very low sperm count and, although it was just possible for Katy to conceive naturally, it was very unlikely to happen.

Having considered their options and listened to advice, the couple decided to try IVF (in-vitro fertilization) treatment. They knew it would be expensive and they also knew that there was no guarantee that the treatment would succeed on the first occasion. But they had talked it over and were determined to go ahead. After an anxious wait, Katy and Jack were overjoyed to discover that all had gone well and that Katy was indeed pregnant.

For the first 12 weeks of the pregnancy Katy was aware of a constant nervousness in case anything should happen to cause her to lose the baby. After that time, however, she felt more able to relax – although she was still careful about diet, rest, and so on. She would spend part of each day relaxing and allowing her mind to conjure up thoughts of what the baby might be like.

And then suddenly, when she was 18 weeks pregnant, Katy miscarried. There was no warning. It all happened in the course of one day and there was nothing anyone could do to prevent it. Katy was devastated. After all she'd been through to become pregnant in the first place, after the care she'd taken and the dreams she'd had, it seemed so cruel to have it all snatched away. The loss was made all the greater by the knowledge that she and Jack would have to go through the IVF treatment again – with all its costs (both emotional and financial) – if they wanted to try for another baby.

For people like Jack and Katy who had spent months thinking about babies before Katy even became pregnant, there is no possibility of looking on the miscarriage as a medical condition. They had lost the baby they so longed for and for whom they had struggled so hard.

But it is equally possible for someone who has a very early miscarriage to feel the loss of her baby – even when logic tells her that the foetus had not yet developed. This sort of person should never be dissuaded from her train of thought but should be allowed to go on following her feelings and letting herself grieve for the child that never was.

Other women, if the miscarriage takes place in the very early stages of the pregnancy, find that they are able to detach themselves completely from all thoughts of an actual baby.

Patsy couldn't have been more than six or seven weeks pregnant when she had a miscarriage. As she told me, 'But for the missed period and the home pregnancy test I used, I probably wouldn't even have known that I was pregnant. I did feel a bit sick on one or two mornings but might easily have put that down to a stomach bug or something similar. I certainly hadn't got around to thinking of a real baby yet – there simply hadn't been time.'

Because of this sense of detachment and because the pregnancy had not been planned, it was easier for Patsy not to think about the loss of a human life when she had her miscarriage.

We have already seen that in the UK the law requires all babies born after the twenty-fourth week (and all those born before that time but able to sustain life outside the womb) to have their birth and death registered and to be buried or cremated. But what of those places where this does not apply or all those babies born before the twenty-fourth week and unable to sustain independent life – what happens to them?

June was only 20 years old when she had a miscarriage in the twelfth week of her pregnancy. Some time later she told me, 'I wondered what "it" was like – I wasn't allowed to see anything – and what they would do with "it" afterwards. I was too scared to ask, partly because I didn't want to appear ignorant and partly because I thought I might not like what I was told. So I just said nothing. Some time later I found out that it was usual for the product of a miscarriage to be incinerated and that really upset me. It made what I had been through and the life I had been carrying inside me seem worthless. I felt very hurt; it appeared to trivialize the whole concept of pregnancy.'

Hospitals vary greatly in what they do after an early miscarriage. Some still incinerate everything but others will carefully separate the foetus from any other material and will use a separate incinerator for this, thereby at least according it some respect.

Rosemary suffered an early miscarriage in a hospital which not only used separate incineration facilities but which held a service in the hospital chapel once a month. Any parents who had lost babies through miscarriage or stillbirth were invited to attend. Rosemary and her partner went along.

I rather dreaded going. In fact I couldn't face it just after I lost
the baby. We finally went about three months later – and I
might not have plucked up the courage then if Andy hadn't
persuaded me. But I'm so glad I went.

It was a lovely service. There were flowers and soft music
and some of the nurses and midwives were there too. I suppose the loss of a baby must be hard on them as well. The
chaplain said some prayers and then spoke to us about
the souls of our babies. I'm not even a religious person really
but I was so pleased that I went even though it made me cry.

They said we could come back again if we wanted and we
decided to go back on the day our baby would have been born
and again a year after I lost her – and by that time I was
already pregnant with my daughter Louise.

If you have an early miscarriage and the hospital in which
you find yourself does not have the facilities for any kind
of memorial service on the premises, you can always
request a burial or a cremation and arrange some type of
memorial service yourself.

All this can be as formal as you wish. If you follow a particular religion, then your minister of religion will help you
plan what you would like to do. Even if you are not
religious, it can be extraordinarily comforting to have a particular spot where the remains or ashes of your baby are
buried and which you can mark with a stone or a plaque.
We all know that, whatever our beliefs, the baby him or herself is not in that place but some people find it beneficial to
have somewhere to go – perhaps with some flowers – when
they feel the need, or perhaps to mark a special anniversary.

Giving the baby you have lost a name – however early
the miscarriage – can also be helpful at such a time. A
name on a plaque or stone makes the baby a true part of
your family, however many other children you may go on
to have.

Perhaps this is a good point at which to stop and reflect
upon what you think happens after we die. Everyone –
whatever their religious upbringing – has their own
personal opinion and, even though in the western world

we do our best never to think or talk about death, it is something we should consider from time to time.

If you are someone who believes that there is nothing at all after this life, at least you have the comfort of knowing that your baby cannot be suffering in any way. This does not make your sadness any less, but the tears are for yourself and for the part of your family that you have lost. That is not wrong. We are all entitled to cry when we are unhappy, but it is good to understand just what we are crying for.

If you believe that there is something after this life – even if you are not really sure what that something is – then your baby is in a better place. Not only that but, when the time comes, you will see him or her again and your family will be complete.

Most people who believe in another life after this one also believe that those who die as babies or children continue to grow to adulthood in this other world. You may find it comforting from time to time to imagine what stage your child has reached. You can still talk to him or her – either aloud or in your head. This is not something about which you should become obsessive and the need to do it will probably grow less as time goes by.

Those who believe in reincarnation – that the spirit passes from one body to another after an interval of years – also believe that the lives we live are all part of a great learning process and that each spirit chooses the family into which it wishes to be born and the lessons it wishes to learn during that lifetime. It is also felt that those who die as unborn babies or as very young children are actually such wise and evolved spirits that they have no need to live another whole life on earth but can progress now to whatever lessons or rewards lie before them in a later world. So, while you are naturally sad at having lost your baby, at the same time you should be proud of the fact that you were chosen as the mother of a being so evolved that he or she only needed to touch this earth long enough to help you to learn something.

In the case of a later miscarriage, most hospitals now have the facility for taking a photograph of the baby and this is given to the mother or the couple concerned. If this is offered to you, I hope you will accept it as, even if you feel that it would hurt too much to look at it now, it can prove a comforting memento at a later date.

Cassie was in her twenty-second week when she lost the baby she was carrying. Because of some complications which arose, she had to have surgery under general anaesthetic immediately afterwards. When she awoke the nurse told her that they had taken a photograph of the baby – a little boy – and offered to show it to her.

At first Cassie was somewhat apprehensive. She was afraid of what the photograph would show and whether the baby would look normal or not. Eventually she plucked up the courage to look at it and was very moved by what she saw. The photograph was of a very tiny but very beautiful baby boy wrapped in a lovely white shawl. He looked perfect and just as though he was sleeping.

Cassie later told me of the various stages of having such a photograph in her possession. In the very early days she carried it everywhere with her and would look at it often, though to do so caused her to weep. Then she went through a phase when she put it in a drawer and could not bring herself to look at it at all. As time passed, however, and the harshness of that early agony abated, she would just take that photograph out from time to time and look at it with sadness but also with love. She was so pleased that she had accepted it in the first place and later, when she had two subsequent children, that photograph was put in the family album and the other children knew that this was their little brother who had died.

There are many ways of commemorating the fact that your baby had a life, however brief. What you choose to do will depend upon your own feelings and also, to some extent, on your financial position. While those who can afford it may choose to make some public donation or gift in memory of their lost baby, others will prefer to make a more private gesture of commemoration. But, almost without exception, everyone I have spoken to seems to find that doing *something* helps them to come to terms with their loss.

Jackie was 17 when she found she was pregnant by a boy she hardly knew. She'd had too much to drink at a party and ended up in bed with a young man she didn't even particularly like. And, as soon as he heard of the pregnancy, he denied all responsibility and would have nothing whatsoever to do with Jackie.

How she dreaded telling her parents. They were fairly puritanical in outlook and her father had quite a temper so she was actually afraid of how they were going to react. In the end she plucked up the courage and, to her surprise, they took it quite calmly and were more supportive than she had expected.

For a short time Jackie considered having an abortion but she didn't really feel that this was something she could bring herself to do. Her father insisted that, once the baby was born, it should be put up for adoption immediately. This was not something Jackie wanted but she was still at school and totally dependent upon her parents. So, in order to keep the peace, she did not argue. Secretly, however, she hoped that, once they had seen what was to be their first grandchild, her parents would not be able to bring themselves to part with the baby.

Then, in the fourteenth week of her pregnancy, Jackie had a miscarriage. She wasn't ill and there was no great pain – just a small amount of discomfort and that was it. She was taken into hospital where she had an ERPC, after which she returned to her parents' home.

The thing which hurt Jackie so much – and which was still causing her such distress two years later that she came to see me for help in dealing with it – was that her parents kept telling her that 'it was all for the best'. Presumably the older couple meant well; of course, they may just have been relieved that there would not be what was to them the shame of their daughter's pregnancy becoming more obvious. But, giving them the benefit of the doubt, perhaps they really were thinking of Jackie and that she would now be able to get on with her education and her life.

But to Jackie – even though she had not intended to become pregnant in the first place – this had been a real baby, *her* baby. How could its loss be 'all for the best'?

Jackie was nearly 20 when she came to see me. She was in her second year at university and still living at home during the vacations. In many respects life was going well for her, but there was always the shadow of the baby she had lost somewhere in the back of her mind. What made things even more difficult was that, from the day of the miscarriage, she'd had no one she could talk to about it. After their 'all for the best' comment, her parents had never mentioned the pregnancy or the miscarriage again – and she had certainly never had the courage to bring the subject up. The only other person who knew what had happened was her doctor and, since Jackie hardly ever saw him, she supposed that the event was now just a comment on her medical notes.

During one of our early conversations I asked Jackie if she had anything to remind her of her baby's existence. She said she had not. I suggested that she try to think of something she could buy which would serve as a tangible memento – something she could take with her from place to place and which would have a special meaning for her, even if other people did not realize this.

When she came to see me the following week, Jackie told me that she had bought a teddy bear in memory of her baby. This teddy bear now sat on the end of her bed and she would just touch it as she wished it goodnight and good-morning. Her parents, not realizing the significance of the toy, had made no comment when she bought it and it was small and portable enough for her to take to university during the term time.

That was a very small way in which a baby's life was commemorated but it brought to the young woman concerned an enormous amount of comfort and helped to heal the wound which had been with her for so long.

Other people find their own ways of marking and commemorating the all-too-brief life of their baby. One popular form of memento is to plant a flower, bush or tree in the baby's name. This can be a lovely gesture but, should you decide to choose it, do remember to select an easy-to-grow and permanent plant. It would be particularly distressing if the plant were to die at some future date. In addition, do bear in mind the fact that you might move home one day and your memento might prove to be too large and cumbersome to transplant although, if it is a shrub, you might well be able to take a cutting with you.

One young woman I spoke to told me that she and her husband planted a Peace rose in their garden after she lost her baby girl. This rose is beautiful, perfumed, strong and hardy and its very name seemed appropriate for the situation. At the same time they had a tree planted in a new woodland area in their daughter's name, knowing that, wherever they might move and whatever might happen to them, that tree would go on for many, many years.

When Shirley suffered a miscarriage in the sixteenth week of her pregnancy, she and her partner Simon decided to sponsor a child in a Third World country by making a monthly donation until that child became an adult. Shirley explained to me that they felt they were giving health and opportunity to a child who would otherwise have been deprived of them and that this was the most fitting tribute to the memory of the child she had lost.

To some people such acts of commemoration might seem to be a morbid preoccupation with their loss. But it is up to the individual mother (or couple) to act in what they feel is the most appropriate way and the one which will bring them the most comfort. There is no right or wrong way to behave when you have lost a baby through miscarriage. Each person must do what they feel the need to do, accepting – as one must after any bereavement – that life goes on and that it would be wrong to allow the loss to colour their entire future. This does not mean that you have to forget – but that you put it in some quiet place at the back of your mind where you can take it out and look at it when you feel the need.

CHAPTER 5

Other People

After a miscarriage the reactions of other people can play a great part – for better or worse – in the mother's recovery. If their words and deeds are positive and supportive, they can be of great benefit and help as the woman learns to come to terms with the loss of her baby.

Should other people react in a negative way, however, it can serve to increase the despair and despondency the mother is already experiencing, as well as deepen her sense of isolation and loneliness.

At any time of trauma in our lives, we need other people around us – preferably family and friends but also counsellors or members of a support group. Being able to share our pain and grief with others can help to ease the situation, even when those with whom we share it can do nothing but be there for us with a caring word or a sympathetic touch.

The trouble is that most people find it very difficult to deal with a bereavement of any kind and this is even more the case when it is not only a baby who has been lost, but a baby who has never had a life outside the womb. They do not know what to do or what to say. But they are needed nonetheless – even if all they do is provide a hand to hold or a shoulder to cry on.

Marie told me that she felt like two people when faced with this situation after her second miscarriage. 'One part of me could understand how difficult my friends found it to say or do anything to help – I could even sympathize with them in a way. But the other part of me – the part with shattered emotions – just wanted them to be there.'

Of course it is possible for those close to the woman to say or do the wrong thing and thereby make the situation worse. Many of the women I interviewed when preparing to write this book felt that their hurt and distress had been compounded by the words or the attitudes of other people. Some felt that the very existence of their baby had been trivialized.

Lizzie, who had lost her baby in the tenth week of her pregnancy was told by her (well-meaning) sister-in-law that she was lucky the miscarriage had occurred so early on before she'd had time to get attached to the baby. Lizzie was furious. How dare she say that! This was *her* baby and, however brief the pregnancy, of course she had become attached to it.

Paula's aunt told her that she could 'always try again', adding that 'At least you have Thomas.' Paula couldn't believe her aunt could be so insensitive. She loved her little boy and she would love any other children she might have in the future, but that made no difference to the fact that she also wanted the baby she had lost.

Some people – even close members of the family – find any talk of loss or death so uncomfortable that they try to carry on with life as though nothing has happened.

Jeanne's family had never been particularly demonstrative, finding it difficult to put their feelings into actions or words. When Jeanne came home from hospital, having had a miscarriage, no one mentioned the subject at all. Various people asked her how she was or if she was 'feeling better', but it was as if the baby had never existed. Jeanne began to feel that she had to put on an act and become a bright, positive young woman who did not have a care in the world.

We all have our different ways of grieving but, however we do it, the process is important. Some women, after a miscarriage, will want to talk about what has happened while others simply want a sympathetic shoulder to weep on and a sympathetic ear to listen. Some women will exhibit an almost overwhelming sense of grief while others will carry with them a quiet air of intense sadness. It is up to those who are the friends or relatives of such women to follow their lead and, putting aside their own natural tendencies, to allow them to work through their loss at their own pace. It is often hard to realize just how long this process can take and how important it is to maintain contact for as long as necessary.

In the case of Jeanne and her unemotional family, the person who made all the difference was a neighbour who lived a couple of doors away. In the early days she would come to the house and quietly help Jeanne to get on with the practical chores involved in caring for her home. Together they would tidy, dust or wash dishes. When Jeanne needed to talk, this new friend would listen; when she was lost in her own thoughts, nothing was said.

Jeanne told me how much comfort she got from this woman's presence. Even some months later, there would be a knock at the door every now and then and there would be her neighbour with a bunch of flowers from her garden – 'Just thought you might like these'; or a plate of food – 'I was making a meat pie for us so I made one for you too.'

Because words of sympathy can feel so inadequate, the greatest gift anyone can give someone who has just suffered a miscarriage is to listen. Let her talk about what has happened, about her sadness and about her fears. Talking is so important after a miscarriage because, as there may be nothing tangible to show to prove that the pregnancy ever occurred, it seems to validate the baby's existence.

Rachel told me how much she appreciated the way two of her friends never gave up on her but allowed her to talk to them as much as she wanted. At times she was afraid that she would bore them but they stayed with her and eventually the need to talk about what had happened seemed to lessen and Rachel felt able to face the world and the future again.

The interaction between the woman and her partner following a miscarriage is very important. In some respects the loss of the baby can be just as hard on the man as on the woman. In other ways, however, it can never be quite the same for him as he has never carried the baby within his body.

Abigail's husband was away on business when she had a sudden miscarriage so the fact that he was not physically there for her was not his fault. He came rushing to her side as soon as he heard there were problems but everything happened so quickly that by the time he arrived it was all over.

The first time I saw Abigail she said, 'If Graham tells me one more time that he understands how I feel, I'll scream. *He* wasn't there when it all happened, *he* never felt the baby move inside him – how can he understand? Grieve, yes. Be supportive, yes. But understand how I feel – never!'

The period following a miscarriage can be a very difficult time for men too. They have also lost a baby so, in most cases, they will also be experiencing real grief and sorrow. But because they were helpless to do anything to prevent the situation and because they often feel helpless afterwards, they can feel themselves to be excluded from the whole grieving process.

Some men are just not good at showing their emotions or even at talking about how they feel. Others will do all they can to hold their emotions in check because they are afraid they will upset the woman more if they allow her to see their own grief.

In such cases the best thing for the man to do is to hold his partner and allow her to rant, rave, scream or cry – whatever she feels the need to do. Equally, if she just wants to be quiet or to talk, let her do this. Never rush her, but allow her to take her own time before she is able to contemplate the future again.

When Irene came home from hospital after suffering her second miscarriage, her partner Stuart did all he could to be supportive to her. Thinking he was doing the best thing, he decided to act in a positive and optimistic way, trying to talk to Irene about the future they were going to share and the babies they were going to have some day. But for Irene all this was far too soon; at that stage all she wanted to think about was the baby she had lost. Because she believed that Stuart was no longer interested in that baby, she found it harder and harder to talk to him at all as time went on. Had it not been for the fact that they decided to go for counselling together, their relationship could have broken under the strain.

In those cases where the woman finds it difficult – if not impossible – to talk to anyone, even her partner, and keeps everything bottled up within her, not only is she storing up problems for herself in the future, but she is endangering the partnership by shutting the man out – even though, in the majority of cases, he is suffering too.

The sexual side of the relationship after a miscarriage can also be dramatically affected in a variety of different ways. It is important to avoid sex for at least two weeks in order to avoid any danger of infection. Even after the couple have been told that it is all right for them to resume sexual relations, the woman may not feel emotionally ready to do so. Please don't worry if this applies to you. You are not abnormal – these feelings are quite common – and your former sexual needs and desires will return in time.

Try to explain to your partner how you feel so that he understands what is going on. Also, just because you don't want actual sexual intercourse, it doesn't mean that you cannot share other forms of loving contact with your partner. If even these seem beyond you for a while, there is nothing to stop you telling him of your feelings for him – not to mention the reassurance you will get when he tells you of his for you. Nevertheless, however understanding your partner may be, there may come a time when his sexual frustration causes a rift between you.

Some women go the other way entirely and are so determined to become pregnant again as soon as possible that they want sex at every opportunity. Or else they become so involved in checking dates and temperatures in an effort to ensure that they have the best chance of conceiving again, that all the love and emotion is taken out of the sexual side of the relationship and the man often goes on to feel that he is little more than a 'baby-making machine', which can cause extreme resentment on his part.

Apart from the breakdown this can cause in the relationship, it is a recognized fact that the greater the level of stress and tension, the less likely the woman is to conceive. And checking dates and becoming despondent at the onset of each period can only be stressful. As you will see when you come to the self-help part of this book, the more relaxed you can be about the situation, the more likely you are to conceive again.

A partner's support can be invaluable as time goes on and everyone else has drifted back to their own lives, but grief and sorrow still rear their heads from time to time.

As one woman told me, 'My partner was wonderful; he was the only one I could be totally honest with about the way I was feeling – even months after the miscarriage when everyone thought I had "got over it". I was pretty well OK but every now and then it would hit me – perhaps when I was watching some weepy film depicting family love and closeness or perhaps when the date came round when our little girl should have been born. He never actually said much but he would put his arms around me and hold me tight while I sobbed.'

Sometimes, while the woman is in a highly emotional state after a miscarriage, she may feel that she has let her partner down and that, had he decided to live with someone else, he would have had children by now. Because she may not find it easy to put this into words, it takes a sensitive man to realize what she is thinking and to reassure her that he chose to spend his life with *her* because of the person she is and not because of the children she might eventually bear him.

A man often finds himself in a no-win situation when his partner asks him how *he* is coping after the loss of their baby. If he were to say that he is coping well, he lays himself open to accusations of heartlessness, whereas in reality he might just be trying to be strong for her sake. If, however, he were to break down and sob with her, she might accuse him of prolonging the agony and making the situation – and therefore her – worse.

And, while we all appreciate that the man has not been through the physical experience of the miscarriage in the same way as the woman, it is very hard to stand by and see someone you love in pain and distress – particularly when the miscarriage has taken place over a prolonged period. In addition, because there is often a considerable loss of blood, it can be very difficult to be the one standing by. Most men will know their partner well enough to realize whether she would want him to show his distress or to be the rock for her to lean on. If he is in any way unsure of what she wants, he should understand that the most important thing is for him to be there with her, to try and speak to her of his feelings and to reassure her of his love for her.

Some men are not very good at coping with the physical side of the miscarriage but they stay by the bedside for the sake of their partner. They can have a very tough time watching the person they love in pain, worrying about what is happening and grieving for the baby whose life is ending before it has properly begun.

Sometimes the husband or partner will see the fact of the miscarriage as 'hiccup' in the process of acquiring a family and this can cause them to feel disappointed at the loss of the baby, rather than grief-stricken, which might be difficult for the woman to understand. In fact, she may begin to think that he doesn't care at all and so the marriage could become severely threatened.

A mother who has suffered a miscarriage may also have one or more other children to take into consideration.

Many people tend to think of miscarriages as happening during the first pregnancy or of one woman suffering many miscarriages and being unable to have children at all. But this is far from the case. Although probably less common, it is far from rare for a woman who already has children to have one or more miscarriages for which no explanation can be found.

How you deal with existing children after you have had a miscarriage depends very much upon the age of the children concerned and the stage of pregnancy which had been reached.

If the miscarriage is an early one, it is quite possible that nothing will yet have been said to other children in the family. But if the pregnancy is well advanced then older children will certainly be aware of what is happening and young ones might have been told that 'there is a baby in Mummy's tummy' or 'you are going to have a little brother or sister'.

Once that stage has been reached, you are going to have to find some way of telling those children about the loss of the baby – and trying to do so without frightening them about what might happen to any future babies or about the health of their mother.

It is always best, when discussing any sort of bereavement with children, to be as honest with them as you can – naturally bearing in mind their age and the level of their understanding. Nor should you try to hide your own grief from them; what has happened is a sad occurrence and they need to understand that you are unhappy about it. But reassurance is also necessary, both regarding the fact that this doesn't happen to every pregnancy and regarding your own health. You may well have spent time in hospital and, to a child, any sign of illness in their mother can be very frightening.

Kate hadn't intended this pregnancy to happen at all. She and her husband already had four children; the two boys were in their early teens and the two little girls were aged two and four years. She had never had any problems either in conceiving or during pregnancy with any of those children. But, just as she was getting used to the idea of having a fifth child, she had a miscarriage and was amazed to find how distressed she was.

The two boys knew about the pregnancy from the beginning but it was early days and the little girls had not yet been told. Kate was surprised to find that her sons were really upset about what had happened and were extremely concerned about their mother and her health.

When I spoke to Kate some weeks after her miscarriage, she told me that the boys had played a major part in helping her to come to terms with what had happened. If she felt she needed to cry, they were there to put their arms around her and give her all the comfort they could. If she wanted to talk about what had happened, they were ready to listen to the same facts over and over again. Ever protective of their little sisters, the boys would take the girls off Kate's hands whenever they sensed that she was feeling distressed but did not want the little ones to become aware of it.

The other thing which surprised Kate was that, the pregnancy not having been a planned one and having thought her family complete with the four children she had already, she found herself yearning for another baby. Her husband was quite amenable to the idea and, four months after I saw her, she was once again pregnant. This time all went well and the following year she gave birth to an eight-pound baby boy.

One of the things Kate told me was that, far from finding it an extra strain telling her teenage sons about the miscarriage, it was their love and support which helped her to come to terms with what had happened more quickly than she might otherwise have done.

You might think that the one person a woman should be able to turn to after a miscarriage would be her mother – and in many cases this is so (and mothers-in-law can be pretty good too). But, if the mother concerned has never been a particularly warm or caring person, the fact of the miscarriage is not going to suddenly turn her into one.

A mother who has always found it difficult to talk to her daughter about the onset of periods, about sex or any other intimate subject is likely to find it just as difficult to find the right words to say if that daughter suffers a miscarriage. This doesn't necessarily mean that she doesn't care or isn't truly distressed but, if she is someone who finds it difficult to demonstrate such emotions, she is probably not the one you should look to for comfort now.

In some ways the loving mother is in the same position as the partner; she also has to stand by and see you suffer and this is never easy. And, while of course it is not her baby, nonetheless it can be immensely comforting to talk to her just because she is a woman who has had children herself.

Caroline thought that her mother would be just the person to turn to after she had her miscarriage. After all, she had had two miscarriages herself before the births of Caroline and her sister. And yet she got little comfort from that quarter. Her mother's attitude was quite brusque and Caroline was harshly informed, 'I got over it so it's about time you did.'

You know your own mother – the type of person she is and whether she is able to communicate on personal topics like this. You are not going to change anyone now so, if you think she would not be the right person for you to turn to, listen to those inner feelings. If, however, you feel that she would be helpful, comforting and understanding, then your mother could well be the person to give you the greatest help at a difficult and distressing time.

A woman who has had a miscarriage will have her emotions in a turmoil and may be surprised at some of the feelings she experiences with regard to her friends. Here are just a few of the things I was told when I was interviewing women for this book:

'For ages I couldn't bear to see a pregnant woman. And it seemed as though every woman I looked at in our town was pregnant. I hated myself for feeling this way but I just couldn't help it.'

'My best friend had an abortion when she was much younger. I've always known about it and it has never bothered me. But suddenly, after the miscarriage, I couldn't bear to be in the same room as her – I felt as though I hated her and the feeling really frightened me. It passed eventually and everything is all right now but it was really scary at the time.'

'I found it very difficult to take my little girl to nursery school because everyone there knew I had been pregnant and knew I'd had a miscarriage. I felt as though they were all looking at me and wondering what was wrong with me (though I don't suppose they were really). I wanted to scream at them and tell them that I wasn't a freak, just someone who had lost a baby.'

'It was a real effort to sound pleased for my younger sister when she phoned and told me that she and her husband were expecting their second baby. *Second* one – she's three years younger than me and I hadn't even been able to carry one to full term. I tried to say the right things but I know that inside me there was this horrible person who almost hoped that she'd lose her baby too.'

All the above are direct quotes from women who are kind, loving and caring but who, as part of their bereavement process, experienced these negative feelings which were totally alien to their usual way of thinking. The reason for quoting them here is to show you that this sort of thing is a normal part of grieving – so please don't be alarmed if you find yourself experiencing such thoughts. They will pass in time and you will return to being the person you always were.

A woman who has suffered a miscarriage needs to know herself and whether she is the type of person who would find comfort in a support group or whether she prefers to talk to someone on a one-to-one basis – whether that someone is a friend, a relative or a professional counsellor.

Some women feel they only want to talk to others who have had the same experience. Others prefer a professional who cares about them but who is one step away from the situation. Just remember that talking is an essential part of the healing process and, whichever method you choose, it helps to realize that what you are experiencing is normal.

CHAPTER 6

Help and Self-help

The miscarriage has happened. It is a fact. Nothing any-one says or does can change it now. All that can be done – and all that should be done – is to work to deal with the trauma, overcome any residual problems and look towards the future in the most positive way possible.

This chapter and the next two are designed to help you to do just that. In this chapter you will find explanations of techniques you can use to help yourself as well as details of one organization and practitioners who may be able to assist you too. (All necessary addresses will be found in the reference section at the back of the book.)

In Chapter 9 we will go together through each stage of the miscarriage and its aftermath and explore the most effective ways of dealing with what has occurred.

Let's begin with a very important UK organization which has already been mentioned in this book.

THE MISCARRIAGE ASSOCIATION

This organization has been in existence since 1982 when it was founded by a group of women, each of whom had personal experience of miscarriage. From these quite humble beginnings, the United Kingdom now has more than 200 volunteer telephone contacts and 80 support groups.

To quote their literature:

> The Miscarriage Association is a national charity which provides support and information for all on the subject of pregnancy loss. We gather information about causes and treatments and promote good practice in the way pregnancy loss is managed in hospitals and in the community.

The Miscarriage Association can help you in various ways: it can put you in touch with a telephone volunteer in or near the area in which you live; it can tell you how to contact your nearest support group so that you can get together with others who have also suffered pregnancy loss. There you will be able to talk with people who you know can understand what you have been – and are – going through.

Don't think that such meetings are either morbid or negative. Although everyone present has been drawn there by the common bond of miscarriage, there is much that is positive too. Some groups have talks by caring professionals who are able to offer helpful advice and hope, and there may also be visits from members who have gone on to enjoy successful pregnancies and can therefore give encouragement to those who may still be in the early stages of their loss.

The Miscarriage Association also publishes a quarterly newsletter as well as up-to-date leaflets and fact-sheets about miscarriage, its possible causes and the treatments currently available. Among its members are professionals who are concerned with the way miscarriage is managed in hospitals and in the community as a whole and, because of this, the organization is working in many ways to promote good practice in those areas.

SELF-HELP TECHNIQUES

1. Relaxation

While I appreciate that relaxation is extremely difficult immediately after suffering a miscarriage, there are many reasons why it is one of the most useful techniques you can learn.

- Because tension in the muscles actually increases the amount of physical pain experienced, learning to relax can reduce the pain and discomfort suffered during or after the miscarriage.
- At times of stress – and what can be more stressful than the loss of a longed-for baby – we are all likely to fall victim to any number of complaints from the relatively minor (such as headaches, insomnia, etc.) to the really serious (such as high blood pressure, strokes and heart-attacks). Stress can be measurably reduced by the repeated practice of an effective relaxation technique.
- Relaxation – particularly when combined with a guided visualization – can help greatly when it comes to dealing with the mental and emotional stress caused by the occurrence of a miscarriage.
- Most treatments given, whether by an orthodox doctor, midwife or nurse or by a practitioner of a complementary therapy, are more effective when the recipient of that treatment is able to relax sufficiently.
- Relaxation is an essential first stage in the practice of visualization which, in itself, can be a positive aid to success in any area of life.
- A relaxation technique is something which can be learned by anyone at all – and learned quite quickly too, although, if it is to be most effective, it should be practised over a period of time. For this reason, those women who feel that they have been somewhat overtaken by events will now be able to reassure themselves

that they are doing something positive towards overcoming their problems.

The Technique

There are many different relaxation techniques, each of which is valid and effective in its own way. If you have ever been to a class in yoga, you will probably have learned one there. But, if you have never been taught a relaxation technique before, then this one will prove simple to learn and will achieve all that you need.

Many people have the wrong idea about relaxing, thinking of it as 'not working' or 'sitting in front of the television'. But it is possible to be doing either of those things and still to be suffering from stress and tension. Real relaxation is something which can be learned and, once you have acquired the skill, will prove highly beneficial at many different times of your life.

A relaxation technique should contain all the following elements.

- You should feel comfortable.
- Your eyes should be closed, to prevent your mind being distracted by the light or by any of your surroundings which might catch your eye.
- Your muscles should be as relaxed as you can make them. A good way of achieving this is to tense them first as it has been shown that, the more you tense a muscle, the greater the contrasting relaxation when you release that tension.
- Your breathing should be even and regular. If you think how, when we are anxious, nervous or stressed, our breathing becomes short and sharp (and, in extreme cases, we hyperventilate), it makes sense to link slow and steady breathing with a calmer and more relaxed attitude.

• Your mind should be occupied with pleasant images. You will find that some relaxation teachers try to insist that you 'make your mind a blank' but – unless you have been practising meditation for years – you are likely to find this impossible and all those worrying or stress-inducing thoughts are likely to force their way in; far better to fill your mind with thoughts and images that you find pleasant as, since we are unable to think of more than one thing at a time, this will effectively shut out all those negative thoughts.

The Setting

Choose a time of day when you have ample time to practise your relaxation technique without watching the clock – you only need about 15 or 20 minutes but, until you are really familiar with the exercise and can do it easily at will, you should practise it every single day if it is to be effective.

The room you practise in should be warm enough to be comfortable, but not so hot or stuffy that you feel uncomfortable or even fall asleep. Fresh air can be beneficial but make sure that you are not in a direct draught.

Your clothing, too, should be comfortable – sufficiently warm to ensure that you don't become chilled and with no tight waistbands or collars to constrict you.

Arrange not to be disturbed while relaxing. If there is someone else around, ask them to answer the door or the telephone; if not, just take the phone off the hook and pretend you're not at home.

Some people like to have gentle music playing in the background while they relax – this is entirely up to you. But, if you do choose to play music, make sure there are no words to interrupt the train of lovely thoughts you might be having.

You may wish to sit in a chair or you might prefer to lie down – on a sofa, the bed, or even the floor. It really makes no difference provided you feel comfortable and that your head and neck are supported (so, if it is a chair, make sure that it has a high enough back or that you have extended it with cushions).

In a moment I am going to give you an actual script which you can use to help you relax. As time goes by you might choose to alter this script to suit your personality and what you like to imagine – but, until that time comes, you can be assured that this particular script works with anyone who uses it, so it makes a pretty good starting point.

Because there is a script and because it is impossible to relax while holding the book in one hand and trying to read from it, there are various things you can do.

- Ask a friend or a partner to read the words to you while you follow what is being said.
- Make a cassette of your own voice, reading the words of the script – but do ensure that you speak very slowly – probably far more slowly than you would have thought necessary; the more we relax, the slower our reactions to what is said to us.
- Use a professionally-produced relaxation cassette. You may already have one but, if not, you will find details of how to obtain one in the back of the book.

When you read the script through before starting, you will see that an image has been used of walking in the countryside as this is something most people can relate to. If, however, this is something you would not like to do in real life, feel free to substitute whatever environment most appeals to you – perhaps a sunny beach, a garden, a mountain slope, a river bank . . . or anywhere that you would find beautiful, pleasurable and a good place to unwind.

The Script

Sit or lie comfortably with your head and neck supported, your legs uncrossed and your hands lying idly in your lap or by your sides. Close your eyes.

Tense the muscles in your feet as tightly as you can . . . and then let them go limp, all at once, so that your feet feel really heavy and relaxed.

Now do the same with your legs and your thighs: tense them and then let them go, let them relax.

Now concentrate on your hands and screw them up into tight fists; hold it for about five seconds and then let them go limp – don't worry if your hands begin to tingle or to feel warm as this is quite normal.

Do the same with your lower and upper arms. Feel the tension in the muscles before allowing them to relax as completely as possible.

Now turn your attention to the whole of your body. Make the muscles in the trunk of your body become tense and rigid and then release that tension so that they are limp. Imagine that your body is growing heavier and heavier with every breath you take.

Now it is time to concentrate on that area where the build-up of tension is usually the greatest – your shoulders, head, neck, face and jaw. Clench your jaw, frown, tense your shoulder muscles so that your shoulders rise towards your ears. Now let all the tension go and be aware of the contrast as you do so. Let your shoulders become relaxed and heavy; let your jaw relax; even allow your eyelids to feel heavy.

Now spend some time concentrating on your breathing. Let it become even and regular – concentrate on the rhythm of your breathing. When it is really steady, just breathe in and out ten times, counting in your head as you do so.

Next it is time to use your imagination to take you to a place which you would find beautiful.

I'd like you to imagine that you are standing in a country lane, looking around you at the beautiful scenery there. Put into that picture whatever you would most like to see – this is your lane and the view is your view.

Perhaps you can see fields of grass or of wheat with a backdrop of hazy purple hills. Perhaps there are cattle in the fields or sheep on those hills. You might see farms or cottages. There may be a river or a stream with water reflecting the light from the sky above. Take your time and allow the picture to develop in your mind – changing things whenever you wish – until you reach what is to you the perfect image.

Spend a few moments allowing this image to fix itself in your mind so that you can go there again whenever you wish. Make sure that you know what it looks like from every angle and what it feels like to be there.

Now start to saunter slowly along that lane, looking to the right and the left and taking in the beauty of the scenery your mind has created. It is a lovely day, warm and sunny but not too hot and with just enough of a gentle breeze to keep the temperature pleasant. Feel the sun on your face and your arms, feel the breeze just brushing against your hair. Listen to the sounds around you: rustling of leaves, the song of the birds in the trees, the gentle lowing of a cow in a nearby meadow . . . Breathe deeply and absorb the fresh green smells of the countryside on a lovely day.

Walk along that lane for a while, looking to the right and left and enjoying what you see. Eventually you come to the edge of a small wood – this is not a frightening place but somewhere cool, soft and inviting. The trees there are straight and strong and very, very old.

In your mind, stretch out your hand and touch the trunk of one of those old, old trees. It's warm and rough and crinkly, and you can feel the energy pulsating through it.

Walk on into the wood now. The ground is softer; it's a quiet and peaceful place. It is a little darker here as the leaves of the trees meet high above your head, but just ahead of you is one spot where the sun is shining through – where the leaves of the trees don't meet above your head.

Go forward to that patch of sunlight and stand in it. Feel the rays of the sun washing over you like a warm shower, easing away any accumulation of stress and tension, leaving you feeling calm, strong and very, very relaxed.

Picture a cat; think how a cat stretches in the sun, just for the joy of it. Imagine yourself doing just that – reaching up and stretching so that the sun's rays can touch every part of you, washing away all that stress, all that tension, leaving you feeling so very relaxed.

After a few minutes turn and start to walk out of the wood again, retracing your earlier steps. Your step is a little lighter, your shoulders a little straighter, your breathing a little easier and you feel good.

When you come to the edge of the wood, step out into the bright sunlight of the lane, walking back along the path on which you travelled earlier.

When you reach the point from which you started, stop and take the time to look around you. Take in the beauty of the scenery your mind has created. It is very beautiful, it's yours and you deserve it – so enjoy it.

Know that, whenever you feel the need or desire, you can return in your imagination to this beautiful place and that, whenever you do so, you will be aware of a feeling of deep relaxation and freedom from tension.

Now just take three deep breaths and then, when you feel like it, open your eyes.

No one is trying to pretend that relaxation alone is a cure-all for everything you are feeling after what you have been through. But it certainly helps you to feel better in yourself and to start on your journey to a more positive future.

You can practise the relaxation technique as often as you feel the need. You won't suddenly feel like a new and less stressed you. In fact, it may take three or four days before you notice more than a brief temporary result. But I promise you that, provided you persevere with the practice, you will begin to lose that extreme tension which has been surrounding you and, once you have reached that point, you can be assured that your mind and body are prepared to heal themselves from the trauma they have suffered.

Probably the ideal time to practise a relaxation technique is in bed at night just before going to sleep. This is because, by allowing your mind's last conscious and subconscious thoughts before sleep to be relaxed and positive ones, it is those thoughts which will predominate while you sleep – and you are likely to wake up in a much more positive frame of mind.

(If you choose to keep your practising for last thing at night, you may like to omit the instruction to count to three and open your eyes from the script or the cassette you decide to use.)

2. Visualization

Visualization is just another way of saying 'seeing pictures in your imagination' and it too has great value when it comes to self-healing and to becoming a more positive person.

You may already have heard or read of the way visualization has helped other people. There have been many books and articles on the subject – from the sportsman or woman who 'sees' themselves winning the contest before it begins and who goes on to do so, to the child suffering from cancer who imagines an army of 'good blood cells' fighting the bad ones in their body and then goes on to recover completely from the condition.

Visualization can work for you or against you. We all know of people who, although competent drivers, fail their test time after time through what they think of as 'nerves'. In reality, because they dread the driving test so much, such people tend to tell themselves such things as 'I *know* I'm going to fail' or 'I always hit the kerb when I do a three-point turn.' And, rather as though they had programmed an inner computer, this is just what happens.

I have been using visualization methods to help people get through such things as examinations, driving tests and job interviews for years now with great success. Of course they also need to know what they are doing; they won't pass that test if they have never sat behind the wheel of a car, nor will they pass their exams if they never do any revision. But those are not the usual reasons for failure.

You may wonder what all this has to do with you and the fact that you have suffered a miscarriage (or even more than one). No amount of visualizing is going to bring back the baby you have lost, but it will help both your mind and your body to attain that state of positivity which will enable you not only overcome the past but face the future.

Why does visualization work? It works because the sub-conscious mind is far more receptive to pictures than it is to words. After all, pictures were there first. When you were a little baby in your pram you may have seen a bright red ball on the floor. You liked the look of that ball and knew that you wanted it, but you had no vocabulary and couldn't tell anyone that this was what you wanted. So you may have stretched out your arms to the ball, you may have made noises, you may even have cried for it. Entirely without words, you accepted the knowledge that you really wanted that ball, and entirely without words, you knew that you were happy when someone picked it up and gave it to you.

As we grow up and learn to speak, words – rightly – become very important. As small children we also retain the ability to imagine very clearly (some call it fantasizing, some will say daydreaming, but what are daydreams if not use of the imagination?)

Then, as we grow even older, we often find that our minds become so full of words and facts that we lose the skill of visualizing – some people even see it as a waste of time and effort. And yet it is probably the single most valuable tool for good that you possess.

Suppose you are one of those people who thinks that they are not able to see imaginary pictures in their mind – what then? How are you going to make use of this wonderful tool?

You can rest assured that the only people who cannot imagine in pictures are those who were born blind (and there are other, special techniques to help such people, using their own particular skills). But anyone who has ever been able to see is capable of visualizing. It is a fact, how-ever, that many people temporarily lose this facility as they grow up – whether because of the way in which they were educated or because their lives have become so full of purely practical things that perceived indulgencies, such as flights of fancy, have been discarded.

Think of loss of imaginative ability as a muscle which has grown weak through lack of use. If this had happened to a muscle in your body, you know perfectly well that gentle and repetitive exercise, increasing in strength, would bring the proper ability back to that muscle. The 'muscles' of the imagination are no different. Even if you feel that you can't 'see' anything, practice and repetition will soon enable you to do so.

If this applies to you, follow the four-step routine described below until you feel that you have regained the power of your imagination. It isn't time wasted, I can assure you. The skills of visualization will stand you in good stead, not only at this particular and difficult moment of your life, but at any time in the future when you feel you want to take greater charge of your own destiny.

Improving Visualization

A. Place an object on a table in front of you. Something simple – perhaps a cup, a jug, a vase or even a single flower. Look at that object, observing all you can about it. Don't just think 'that is a vase' – really *look* at it. Notice its shape, its size, its colour. What makes it different to any other vase? Now close your eyes and try to picture that vase in your imagination.

You may find this difficult at first – particularly if you are not used to doing it – but remember that this is not a test. If you are not sure about the appearance of the vase, open your eyes and have another look before then closing your eyes and trying again to picture it. Continue with this exercise daily until you find that task easy.

B. Now move on to a bigger subject. Look at the room in which you are sitting. What can you see from your current position? Once again, close your eyes and try to recreate that scene in your imagination – opening your eyes and having another look if you need to.

C. Once stages one and two come relatively easily to you, repeat the same exercise using another room with which you are familiar but which does not constitute your present surroundings. Perhaps an office in which you work or your bedroom at home. Do exactly the same as you have previously done.

D. The final stage is to visualize an object which is created entirely by your imagination. Picture a scene which would give you pleasure. Create a room, a landscape or a garden in your mind and, when you are happy with it, spend some time there getting to know it – just as if it were a real place.

   Once you can achieve the desired result in all four stages, you will have exercised your 'visualization muscles' sufficiently to help you both now and in the future. In Chapter 8, I will endeavour to show you how you can use this to your advantage at various stages after suffering a miscarriage.

CHAPTER 7

Complementary Therapies

There are now any number of expert complementary therapists who will do all they can to help you at each stage you experience during and after a miscarriage.

I think it is important to note the term 'complementary therapy', as opposed to what some people call it, which is 'alternative therapy'. The latter supposes that you must make a choice between the advice given to you by your doctor, your midwife or your consultant and that given by the therapist. This does not have to be the case at all. It is quite possible for orthodox and complementary medicine to go hand in hand and, indeed, for one to noticeably enhance the other.

Of course, there are some people who insist on consulting *only* a complementary practitioner or *only* their doctor. While it is not for me to deny anyone the right to make their own choices in this as in any other matter, I cannot help thinking that it must be better to examine all the options and then follow the ones which feel right to you.

In this chapter I am going to give you information about the various complementary therapies which may be available to you and what you can expect from them.

Make use of the complementary therapies which are available to you in the physical aftermath of the miscarriage. Several of them can help you to build up resistance to possible infection while, at the same time, treating you in such a way that you achieve a positive hormonal balance as soon as possible.

Complementary therapies may also help with your emotional condition after the miscarriage. An aromatherapist, while giving you a massage which will help you to relax and to lose some of the tension which necessarily surrounds you at such a time, will be able to blend particular oils which are designed to deal with just the emotions we have been looking at.

Bach flower remedies include those recommended for dealing with any or all of the emotions related to bereavement and miscarriage and a specialist will be able to advise you on a specific blend which will help you.

Hypnotherapy will not only help you to relax physically and mentally but will provide you with an opportunity to release from your subconscious all the fears, doubts and anxieties which you may be hiding from others – and even from yourself. And, since most well-qualified hypnotherapists are also counsellors, there will be a chance to discuss the entire situation.

(In all cases you will find in the Complementary Therapists section of this book an organization or address you can contact should you wish to consult a particular therapist.)

ACUPUNCTURE

Acupuncture is an ancient therapy developed over thousands of years in China and other countries of the East. It involves the use of tiny, fine needles on specific points on the body. Although there may be a sensation of some sort (warmth, tingling, etc.) when the needles are inserted just below the surface of the skin, it is not actually painful. The needles are either removed instantly or, in some cases, left there until the end of the session.

As with most complementary therapies, acupuncture takes a holistic and individualistic approach. The practitioner will ask questions about your health, personality and background as he or she works so that, even if two people seek treatment for what is ostensibly the same problem, they will not necessarily be given the same treatment. A very detailed history will be taken and a specific treatment worked out for the individual patient.

Most of the oriental therapies have as their basis the concept of the Chi (Qi) which is the energy force central to the individual. It is when the flow of the Chi is out of balance that problems arise, so the acupuncturist seeks to re-balance it by the treatment given to achieve harmony between the physical, emotional and spiritual elements of the person concerned.

In addition to the use of needles (all of which are sterilized – and you can also request the use of new ones should you prefer), there is sometimes the warming of particular acupuncture points by means of a heated herb, known as moxa.

ACUPRESSURE

This is an ancient form of massage which involves stimulating the acupuncture points with the fingers and thumbs of the therapist. It is sometimes known as 'acupuncture without needles' as it works on the same points and also on the same theory of harmonizing the Chi of the individual concerned.

ALEXANDER TECHNIQUE

The Alexander Technique got its name from its creator, F M Alexander, an Australian actor, who developed the practice in the late nineteenth century. It is based on the theory that only when the body is perfectly aligned does the individual receive efficient muscle feedback – and that lack of such muscle feedback can interfere with the health and the body's ability to function efficiently. The technique aims to help the student's mind and body to work properly together.

Alexander teachers guide their students through various simple physical procedures, giving aid and assistance by verbal instruction and gentle kinaesthetic ('hands on') feedback.

AROMATHERAPY

Aromatherapy usually involves massage with essential oils, blended by the therapist, who will have taken a detailed history from the patient before deciding on the most appropriate oils to be used.

Oils can also be recommended for home use, either in the bath or as an inhalant. These oils are absorbed through the skin and enter the tissues and the bloodstream, thence circulating all around the body. Thus the massage is not only pleasant and relaxing but therapeutic too.

BACH FLOWER REMEDIES

The Bach Flower Remedies were discovered by a medical doctor, Dr Edward Bach, in the 1930s. Dr Bach based his work on the fact that certain flowers had the capacity to heal the body by addressing deep disharmony between the mental and spiritual aspects of our being.

A Bach practitioner, having taken a detailed history from the patient, will create a blend of natural remedies specifically for that patient. The remedies themselves are prepared from natural plants. They come in liquid form and are taken in very small doses; usually they are added in drops to water and sipped at intervals. They work quite quickly on immediate negativity but may take longer to deal with more deep-seated problems.

HERBAL MEDICINE

Herbal medicine, whether Western or Chinese, involves the use of natural plants in the cure of the patient's condition.

As with many other complementary therapies, the herbalist – who will have completed a long training in diagnostic and prescriptive skills – works holistically rather than concentrating on a specific symptom.

HOMEOPATHY

Homeopathy treats like with like, but the remedies are given in such minute doses that, although able to stimulate the body's natural healing ability, they cannot cause side-effects and cannot become addictive. In most cases the remedy is given in tablet form, although there are also powders which dissolve on the tongue and liquids to be taken as instructed.

HYPNOTHERAPY

By helping the patient to relax completely and then by addressing the subconscious mind, the hypnotherapist is able to induce self-healing in that patient.

Many people have misconceptions about hypnotherapy and how it works, believing that they will be 'unconscious', 'out of control' or 'in the power of the hypnotherapist'. This could not be further from the truth. Although very relaxed, the patient will always be fully aware of everything the therapist is saying and will understand every word. At no time will there be any loss of control or subjugation of will on the part of the patient.

Because the subconscious mind is capable of affecting the body's ability to heal itself as well as inducing a sense of positivity in the mind, those who experience hypnotherapy find themselves rapidly becoming far more positive and experiencing a great sense of well-being, in addition to overcoming any problem they may have had.

NUTRITIONAL THERAPY

The approach of the nutritional therapist is holistic in that he or she will seek to look beyond the symptoms displayed in order to find the imbalance which is causing them. The nutritional therapist will look at the patient's eating patterns and also try to discover whether there are any vitamin or mineral deficiencies present. In some cases there may be a problem with toxins in the body or in the patient's digestive processes. Nutritional therapy can also be used to correct imbalance in the female hormones.

Points to bear in mind when consulting a complementary therapist:

1. Where possible choose a therapist because he or she has been recommended to you or because their name is given to you by one of the bodies mentioned in the Complementary Therapists section of this book. All those organizations will ensure that those whose names appear on their registers have undergone the proper training and are fully covered by professional insurance.
2. Any ethical therapist should be willing to have a free chat with you – lasting ten minutes or so – in order that you can be sure that this is the right type of therapy for you.
3. Don't expect an instant 'cure'. Most complementary therapies work on the holistic principle of healing the entire person, as opposed to orthodox medicine which

tends to give you a treatment which deals with a specific symptom. Give the treatment time to work – your therapist should be able to give you a probable estimate of the time scale involved.

4. Because of the holistic approach, which involves working on the patient's emotional tendencies as well as physical ones, it is important that you are completely honest with your therapist. He or she will be covered by similar rules of confidentiality as those which apply to doctors, so nothing you say will ever be repeated to anyone else. Holding back about your feelings, however, could lead to a misdiagnosis on the part of the therapist.

CHAPTER 8

The Way Forward

Having experienced one or more miscarriages is bound to have an effect on thoughts and feelings about future pregnancies from many points of view.

After going through the periods of denial and then of grieving, each woman (and her partner) has to consider whether to try for another baby and, if so, when to begin.

Sometimes, of course, the choice is not yours. Tests after a series of miscarriages may show that you are unlikely ever to be able to carry a baby to full term – and this must be one of the most difficult things for any woman to be told. It seems to single her out, to make her different to every other woman – unable to do the one thing which should come more naturally than anything else.

Of course this is not so and at any one time there are many women who, for one reason or another, cannot have (or are advised against having) a baby of their own. But, if you have just heard these words spoken to you, you are in no mood to think of those other women, or even to consider the possibility that they exist. It is your world which appears to have been shattered, your dreams which are going to remain unfulfilled and you are the one whose self-esteem is lowered as you start to believe that you are 'different' or even 'inferior' to every other woman.

There are various options open to the woman who has been told that she will never bear a child of her own. Some will consider adoption, fostering or even surrogacy, while others will not wish even to think about any of these things and may decide that, if they are not to have their own child, they will have no children at all.

This is a decision which only the woman and her partner can make – and it should not be made too soon. It would certainly be wrong to commit yourself to any future plans while your emotions are still raw from both the miscarriage itself and the news you have been given.

No one can say when you will be ready even to think about making a decision of this sort. For some the time may arrive quite quickly while others will need months, or even years, to think about it.

The most important thing is not to feel that you are under any sort of pressure when making up your mind about the future. You must do what *you* want, not what well-meaning friends and relatives think is best for you and certainly not what you perceive as 'normal'. Nowhere is it carved in stone that every woman must have children, and to go on to acquire a child by one of those other methods should only be undertaken because you really want it, not because it seems that everyone else has a family.

If you decide that you wish to adopt or foster or to use a surrogate to have your baby, then – and only then – should you seek all the advice you can. Not from family and friends but from those professionals who, while fully equipped to explain to you all the possibilities and all the problems, are aware that it is not their place to offer an opinion as to what you should do and what decision you should make. Your doctor, your consultant, your nurse or groups such as the Miscarriage Association in the UK can give you information about all these possibilities but they will still leave you to make up your own mind in your own time.

For those who have not received this devastating news and for whom there should be no difficulty in going ahead with another pregnancy, there is still the matter of when the optimum time for this will be.

This too varies from one woman to another. Some feel that they want to become pregnant again as soon as they can – not to 'replace' the baby they have lost as this would not be possible, but because their maternal instinct has been aroused by the earlier pregnancy.

Lynne had become pregnant for the first time earlier than she and her partner had originally desired but they had accepted the news quite happily and had begun to look forward to the birth of their baby.

Then, in the seventeenth week of her pregnancy, Lynne suffered a miscarriage for which no physical cause was found. Her doctor used that dreadful phrase, telling her it was 'just one of those things'.

Once she was home and beginning to get over the sense of despair she felt at the loss of the baby, Lynne was almost surprised to find that she had developed a desperate longing to have another one as soon as she possibly could. 'I couldn't tell whether it was a physical thing – you know, my body had begun to get itself ready for the baby it was carrying – or whether it was an emotional state and, having discovered that I was going to become a mother, I really felt a great desire to do so,' was how Lynne explained it to me.

Other women feel that – for both physical and mental reasons – they need a time when they are not pregnant. This is partly to give their bodies time to recover from the hormonal changes and the trauma experienced in the pregnancy and the miscarriage. It is partly to give them time to sort out their tangled emotions and to allow themselves ample time to acknowledge the loss of their baby and to let the anguish subside. It may also give them time to allow the special closeness with their partner that shared grief can bring.

Some couples – particularly those who are able to discuss their feelings openly and who are able to demonstrate the depth of their emotion together – feel that their relationship has been strengthened by the loss they have had to endure. Because this puts the relationship on a deeper and more mature footing than may have been the case before, they sometimes wish to take advantage of this and to share special time together before even contemplating the idea of having another baby.

There is also the danger that, if one partner appears to be in too much of a hurry to rush into another pregnancy, the other one may feel that the lovemaking between them, which should be such a joyous experience, has become mechanical and is only indulged in so that conception can take place. It can damage the confidence of either partner if they feel that they are there only to play their part in the conception of a child rather than because they are special to the other person.

When the time arrives – whenever it may be – for the contemplation of another pregnancy, the woman may find that her feelings about the condition have changed. Her confidence in herself and in the functioning of her body may well have been shaken. At one time she probably thought of pregnancy and childbirth as something within the capabilities of every woman and the most natural and uncomplicated thing in the world. Now, of course, she knows only too well that this is not the case. She may well begin to doubt herself and her ability to do what 'every other' woman appears to be able to do.

When she feels able to entertain the thought of another pregnancy may also depend to some extent on how many miscarriages she has experienced and at what stage in her former pregnancies they occurred.

Sonia had only known that she was pregnant for about two weeks when she had her miscarriage. This was her first pregnancy and, having had it explained to her that it is not all that unusual for a first pregnancy to end in an early miscarriage, she felt almost able to think of what had happened as a medical condition rather than the loss of a baby. It was perhaps for this reason that she was able to accept fairly easily the fact that she was pregnant again about two months later.

Valerie, however, had been almost five and a half months pregnant when she lost the baby boy she was expecting. Although, like Sonia, this was her first pregnancy, she had far more time to become used to the thought of motherhood. She had felt her baby move inside her, had spent time thinking of what he would be like, had chosen a pram and started to decorate a nursery for him. To Valerie, this was her baby – there was no way she could ever think of her pregnancy as some sort of 'medical condition'.

Because she had her unborn son to grieve for, it took Valerie many months before she could even face the thought that there was a decision to be made about future pregnancy. The loss was too great, the pain too sharp for any immediate decisions.

Not only do you need time to come to terms with your loss and work through your grief, your body also has to have time to recover. After all, it has been through the hormonal changes associated with pregnancy and has begun to prepare itself for childbirth – and then it has to cope with the trauma and possibly the physical difficulties of the miscarriage.

Ideally, to build up confidence for the future, you need not only to regain your former state of health but to be in even better physical condition than before. And this applies to both the father and the mother. The sperm which the man is constantly producing takes up to twelve weeks to mature. While immature, the sperm can be adversely affected by the diet and stress in the man, as well as by smoking and excess alcohol; they become poorer in both quality and quantity. It is just as important, therefore, for the man's health and lifestyle to be taken into account before conception takes place.

No one is trying to make out that a miscarriage has to be anyone's fault. Nor that, even if a couple do everything in their power to prepare for a future pregnancy, there can be any guarantee of a successful outcome. But it still makes good sense to try to ensure that optimum conditions prevail even before conception takes place. After all, you would not set out on a mountain walk wearing only a cotton dress and thin sandals. You might succeed, but it is less likely than if you were properly prepared.

Pre-conceptual preparation has to be the most sensible approach. It gives the baby the best possible chance in life and gives more peace of mind to the prospective parents because they know they have done all they can to ensure a safe and healthy conception, pregnancy and birth.

In their literature, the Association for the Promotion of Pre-Conceptual Care, Foresight, states:

THE AIMS OF FORESIGHT
We take all possible steps to ensure that every baby is born in perfect health, free from physical and mental handicap and health problems. Foresight Pre-Conceptual Care embraces three plans of action:

1. To secure optimum health and nutritional balance in both parents before conception.
2. To instigate research aimed at the identification and removal of potential health hazards to the developing baby, especially with regard to the environment.
3. To so present the facts and know-how of Pre-Conceptual Care that prospective parents will be motivated to choose to contribute actively to their family's greater health and happiness.

Foresight was founded in 1978. Its two main objectives are, firstly, to safeguard the health of the unborn child by encouraging effective pre-conception care and, secondly, to promote study on the effect on pre-conception health of various aspects of the environment.

In addition to offering help and advice to *both* prospective parents on such topics as optimum nutrition and problems linked with both smoking and alcohol consumption during pregnancy, Foresight gives information on such matters as allergies, heavy metal pollution, screening for genito-urinary infection, vitamin and mineral supplements and ultra-sound scans.

A newsletter is sent to members three times a year. It is also possible to be put in touch with your nearest Foresight Clinician who will be able to give you detailed individual help and advice.

If a woman has suffered more than one miscarriage – and particularly if she has never given birth to a healthy child – it may take even longer for her to contemplate another pregnancy. Whatever logic and statistics may tell her, she will have lost her trust in the whole conception–pregnancy–childbirth cycle. Also, even if she has been given a clean bill of health and assured that further miscarriage is highly unlikely, it is not possible for anyone to promise her that she will not miscarry again.

We all know that becoming pregnant again – or even giving birth to a much-loved and healthy child – can never replace the child you have lost or the sadness you feel about it. But in some ways it can help put the miscarriage into proportion in your life. It was a sad part of your life and one you would not have wished to happen but it does not have to remain the focal point of it.

It is a common reaction to a miscarriage for the woman to be adamant that that's it, she will not try to become pregnant again. For many, however, that is a spontaneous reaction to the trauma and does not last. Some women, however, having reached a stage where they are able to consider their future calmly and logically and less encumbered by the strains and pressures put on them by others, make a calm and reasoned decision to avoid future pregnancy. This decision is perhaps less difficult for those who have one or more children already.

Josie was 39 years old and already had two little daughters when she became pregnant for the third time. It was a wanted pregnancy and both Josie and her husband Jeremy were delighted. So they were both deeply upset when, at just under 14 weeks, Josie suffered a miscarriage.

Josie was surprised by the occurrence as she had never encountered any problems with her previous pregnancies. She was pleased, however, that the miscarriage happened before they'd had the chance to tell their young daughters about the possibility of a future brother or sister – so there were no difficult explanations to make.

Although this pregnancy had been wanted, Josie decided that she could not face trying again. There were several reasons for this. Although not old, she was aware that, at nearly 40, there were more likely to be problems and she decided that she could not face the uncertainty of taking that risk. In addition, she felt that the anxiety she would experience if she did become pregnant again would be likely to affect not only her but her husband and, indirectly, her two daughters and this was not something she was prepared to have happen. She loved her daughters and her husband and she made a decision that that would be the extent of their immediate family unit.

Annette and Steve, on the other hand, had been trying for years to have a family. Not only had it taken Annette a long time to conceive on each occasion, but she had now suffered three miscarriages and she felt that she just could not go through the whole thing again. The anxiety . . . the waiting . . . the doubts . . . the fears . . . the grief – she'd had enough of all these. She was mentally and physically exhausted and felt that she was losing her identity as an individual in the quest for a family.

Annette and Steve investigated the possibility of adoption, but for various reasons this did not seem to be a viable solution for them. They had no desire to foster a child only to face losing them again when the reason for the fostering came to an end. Finally, after much discussion between themselves and with a counsellor they consulted, they decided that they would try no longer but would opt for a life without children of their own.

As Annette told me:

> I love Steve very much and the troubles we have experienced over this have, if anything, brought us even closer together. But it seems as though we have spent years preoccupied with the thought of whether and how we were to become parents. It was just time to stop – to get off the merry-go-round and think of ourselves for once. After all, we married each other because we wanted to be together, not just because we wanted to have children.

I can't pretend that it isn't a disappointment that we can't have a family or that we wouldn't have preferred things to be different. But it is not the end of the world and we have come to terms with it.

Actually, once the decision was made, I felt as though an enormous burden had been lifted from my shoulders. Making it was hard, but living with it surprisingly easy.

For those women who do decide to try again, some find that, once that decision has been made, they conceive very quickly, while others are surprised that they do not. It is not really difficult to understand when this happens as it is an acknowledged fact that stress and tension can make conception more difficult – and who is going to be more stressed than a woman who has already suffered one or more miscarriages and who is anxious about any future pregnancy?

Mandy had a little boy of nearly five when I first met her. Since his birth she had suffered two miscarriages – each in the early stage of pregnancy. On all three occasions she had conceived almost as soon as she wanted but now, eager to have a little brother or sister for Daniel, nothing seemed to be happening.

She'd had examinations and check-ups and had been told by everyone that there was no physical reason why she should not become pregnant again, but still nothing happened.

Mandy found this very difficult. Each month she would wait in hope, only to have those hopes shattered by the onset of her period. Not only was this a deep disappointment, but it seemed to rekindle memories of the miscarriages with all their sadness. As she told me, 'It was like re-opening an old wound every month.'

The more it happened, the more desperate Mandy became to have another baby. She was only too conscious of the fact that she was growing older and also she was aware that, the longer it took for her to become pregnant, the greater would be the gap between Daniel and his little brother or sister.

Mandy was, not surprisingly, becoming very tense and it was only after we had worked together on helping her to become more relaxed in every way that she eventually conceived – after 14 months of trying. She went on to present Daniel with a beautiful little sister.

Because tension makes conception more difficult, the situation often becomes self-perpetuating. With the disappointment which comes each month, the woman tends to feel more stressed and under increasingly more pressure. This makes her even more tense so that she is even less likely to conceive . . . and so on.

In the self-help section of this book you will have seen details of relaxation techniques and also visualization techniques which I have been using for years with those of my patients who were finding it difficult to conceive (whether or not they had suffered a miscarriage) with great success. Although it is not possible to prove that these techniques alone were responsible for the ensuing pregnancies, they certainly went a long way towards making them possible. In some cases it is possible that the practice of a relaxation technique can actually ward off a threatened miscarriage. If you are trying to prepare yourself for the future conception of another child, then relaxation and specifically designed visualization can help you to be both positive and receptive.

The problems don't even come to an end once the woman is pregnant again. Having experienced a pregnancy before which ended in miscarriage, the emotions this time are totally different. Whereas, before having lost a baby, the slight fears and anxieties which accompany any pregnancy were greatly overshadowed by the joy and excitement felt, this time it is very difficult to be as positive. The expectant mother is likely to run the whole gamut of emotions, from the joy and hope for a child of her own to the fear and anxiety resulting from her previous miscarriage. It is also a time when, however well she may be feeling physically, the memories of what happened on that previous occasion are likely to be rekindled, bringing with them fresh waves of grief for the child she lost.

The most difficult time is probably as she approaches the stage of her pregnancy when that past miscarriage occurred. That is bad enough if you lost your baby in the twelfth week but almost unbearable if it happened at, say, twenty weeks. There is all that time to wait and see if, this time, things will go well.

Donna was pregnant for the second time, having lost her first baby in the fourteenth week of her pregnancy. This time all seemed to be going well – she was in her twentieth week and all scans and examinations were positive. But, as she told me, Donna felt cheated. This should have been a time when she could have experienced the utter joy of expecting her baby and yet, even now, she was scared to hope or to trust her condition. It was, she said, like waiting to slip over on a banana skin. It seemed to her to be so unfair to have been deprived of the opportunity of being happy.

Even when all is going well, pregnancy – and particularly a first pregnancy – is a time of strange physical feelings. There are the movements of the baby within you; you may suffer from such things as wind, backache or constipation. All these things can be part of any pregnancy but, if you have already experienced a miscarriage, every little twinge can frighten you in case it is a sign that everything is going wrong again. If you are experiencing this sort of fear, it is important to remain as calm as possible. So stop what you are doing, take some deep breaths and relax to the best of your ability. See if you can find some logical explanation for the sensations you feel – sensations which quite often disappear spontaneously once you have relaxed. If you are still worried or unsure, telephone your doctor for advice.

It is also likely that the expectant mother will feel quite different when it comes to making preparations for the new baby.

Alison had miscarried her baby daughter in the twenty-second week of her first pregnancy. Until it actually happened she had been feeling quite well and, together with her partner Nigel, had made all sorts of preparations. Baby clothes had been bought and made and neatly put away. Names had been discussed and the small bedroom had been decorated as a nursery.

This time things were very different and Alison found that the only way she could cope was almost to pretend that she wasn't pregnant at all – just that she was going about her ordinary life but happened to be growing larger. She would not let anyone tell her the sex of the baby she was expecting, convincing herself that, should the worst happen, it would not be so bad if she lost 'it' as opposed to 'him' or 'her'.

She would not think about names or which type of pram she would like. And, although the nursery had been newly decorated and never used, Alison felt that it must all be done again as the original decorations had been chosen for the little daughter who never lived to see them.

Having made the decision to act in this way and to avoid 'tempting fate' (as she put it), Alison thought it might make this pregnancy easier to deal with – but it didn't really. Now, in addition to all the other emotions she had to deal with, she felt secretly guilty in case the baby she was now expecting felt unloved or unwanted.

Maggie said that, when she became pregnant after having had two miscarriages, she only went once to the ante-natal classes as she felt like a complete outsider. 'There were all these women,' she said 'assuming that everything would be fine. I couldn't be like them as I had personal experience of how things could go wrong and how devastating that could be. I couldn't tell anyone there how I felt as I didn't want to destroy their confidence or put thoughts of miscarriages into their minds.'

Maggie even felt awkward about continuing to go to meetings of her local group of the Miscarriage Association. 'I know it's stupid,' she told me, 'but I felt embarrassed because I was now pregnant and they were not. Also, just being there kept reminding me of what could happen to me.'

Because it is always good for anyone to be able to talk about how they are feeling, it was extremely fortunate that Maggie discovered by chance that her neighbour – a woman in her fifties with children and grandchildren of her own – had suffered two miscarriages herself when she was young. Now Maggie had someone to talk to who was not only living proof that it is possible to go on to have a family successfully after miscarriages, but who was able to understand just how Maggie herself was feeling in a way that few other people – however kind their intentions – could.

This is a time for each woman to find her own way of balancing her fragile emotions. Some find it easier not to tell anyone – apart from those closest to them – about the pregnancy until it becomes really obvious. It is bad enough to feel that you are walking on eggshells because of what might happen without feeling that everyone else is watching too. Keeping it a secret is all very well but can make things somewhat difficult if you find yourself feeling sick or unwell and unwilling to join in things as before.

Following the superstitious path and refusing to make firm preparations for the baby is also understandable. But, from the unborn baby's point of view, the sooner that loving communication between mother and child is established, the better. Hypnotherapists can prove that babies in the womb are aware of emotions – happy, sad, angry, loving, etc. So it is really important for a loving link to be created at the earliest possible stage even if it makes things harder on the mother should there be another miscarriage. But that must be weighed against the undoubted benefits to the child if – as is to be hoped – all goes well. (You will find more details of how to establish this mother/baby link later in this book.)

Above all, anyone who has been through an experience as traumatic as a miscarriage needs to find someone to talk to – preferably someone who understands what you have been through but who is not too closely involved in your personal life.

Some doctors and midwives are excellent at this while others appear to be harrassed and preoccupied. Here are just a few of the comments made about them by some of the women I interviewed:

- 'My doctor was just wonderful. I must have driven her mad, running to her every time I felt a twinge I did not understand, but she never lost patience with me. She even arranged for me to have an extra scan at one point, just to set my mind at rest.'
- 'I could almost see my doctor sigh as I entered the surgery. He was so patronizing and spoke to me as though I was two years old.'
- 'I got into a panic at one stage because I hadn't felt the baby move for ages. The consultant was really kind and arranged a scan for me almost immediately.'
- 'I'd had two miscarriages in the past but, after the initial consultation and confirmation of my current pregnancy, he just said he would see me again at 18 weeks. I reminded him that I had suffered two miscarriages at about twelve weeks but he said that it made no difference.'
- 'The midwife who looked after me when I was expecting my daughter was the one who had been with me when I had my miscarriage. She was wonderful. She knew how nervous I was and she would phone for a chat and to see how I was. Sometimes she even popped in on her way home from work and spent a few minutes with me, feeling the baby move, listening to the heartbeat and generally reassuring me. I don't know what I would have done without her.'

If you are lucky with those around you and can find someone who will understand how you feel and give you a chance to express your fears before offering reassurance, that is fine. If not, perhaps you could look for a caring professional to talk to – someone who can devote to you the time you need.

CHAPTER 9

Help at Every Stage

1. ARE YOU AT RISK?

It is possible for any woman to suffer a miscarriage but there are certain categories who are more at risk than others and they are listed below. If you fall into one of these categories, please don't worry – it doesn't mean that you are bound to experience a miscarriage or that you cannot have children. The list is simply put here so that you may be more aware of the situation and take more care of yourself during your pregnancy. In addition, should you experience any pain or sensation which you cannot understand, it is more important for you (even though it may turn out to be nothing at all) to seek help or advice.

The higher risk categories include:

- Women whose pregnancy results from fertility treatment. By definition, since fertility treatment was needed in the first place, such women may experience more difficulties during pregnancy than others. It is essential, therefore, that they take extra care of themselves and allow themselves to rest far more.
- Women who are older when they conceive. This applies particularly if they have not yet had any children.

- Those who are expecting twins or the birth of a greater number of babies. Rest is essential for these women, particularly as the pregnancy progresses.
- Those women whose periods began at an earlier age than is usual. It has been shown that such women are more likely to miscarry than those whose periods began later.

What to do

If you fall into one of the above categories – and especially if you have already had a miscarriage – try to take extra care before becoming pregnant again.

Various complementary therapies – such as homeopathy, herbalism and acupuncture – offer a course of treatment designed to put you in the best possible state of health to conceive, carry and give birth to a child.

Aromatherapy can aid relaxation and relief from stress, as can hypnotherapy. The latter also uses visualization and positive thinking techniques, combined with hypnosis, to put you in the right frame of mind for a successful pregnancy.

The organization Foresight will give you information on the ideals of diet and other aids to help both you and your partner be in the optimum condition before conception, thereby giving both mother and baby the greatest chance of health and a successful birth.

2. EARLY SIGNS

Any of the symptoms listed below may indicate that there is a threat of a miscarriage. It will not necessarily be the case that a miscarriage is bound to follow – but, should you experience one or more of these symptoms, you would be well advised to consult your doctor for a check-up. Not only will this confirm that all is well but it will help to put your mind at rest, thus reducing the amount of stress you feel.

- Abdominal pain or a constant backache. Of course, these things may also be due to other causes. It is also possible that you may experience them before you even know that you are pregnant. If you do know, however, please don't ignore them but seek advice as soon as possible.
- Bleeding (especially if the blood is clotted) from the vagina.
- Cramps – somewhat like period pains. Once again, it is possible that you will experience these before you realize that you are pregnant.

What to do

- Call your doctor and then go straight to bed. The doctor will be able to assess the situation but he or she will need your help. You should be ready to tell him or her all you can about the pain or the bleeding. When did it start, how severe is it, is it constant or intermittent? The doctor might want to do a manual examination of the cervix or a urine pregnancy test. Sometimes progesterone will be given if it is felt that this is necessary – a deficiency of this hormone can be one of the causes of a miscarriage.
- You may be taken to hospital, either just for a rest and observation or for the administration of progesterone by drip.
- You should go to bed and stay there, only getting up to visit the toilet. Try to arrange for someone to bring you meals and to keep you company if possible. You will do yourself no good if you spend all your time lying there thinking of the possibility of a miscarriage.

  This type of complete bed rest should make any bleeding stop within about 24 hours. If it does not, contact your doctor or the gynaecological department of your local hospital; you will probably be admitted for observation.

- Try to relax if possible. I know this is much easier to say than to do at such a time but it really can make a difference. Perhaps listening to a relaxation cassette will help you. This is a time when hypnotherapy to help you with visualization and positive thinking – as well as with the relaxation process itself – could be extremely beneficial. It will not make a great difference if you are in a position where the miscarriage is inevitable, but it might well prevent those miscarriages which occur because the excess stress and tension being experienced by the expectant mother play a part in causing it to happen.

- Try to find things to occupy your mind while you are resting physically so that – even if only for short periods at a time – you focus on something other than the fact that you are frightened that you are about to miscarry or that you feel unwell.

  The ideal in such circumstances is to have someone there to talk to as you will have to pay attention to what they are saying in order to reply. But it needs to be someone who is sensitive and understanding enough to realize when you are growing tired and will then keep quiet and allow you to relax.

  If you do not have anyone who can spend that much time with you, try reading, listening to the radio, watching television and doing puzzles in order to keep your mind occupied.

3. FUTURE PREGNANCIES

- If, as a result of medical examination, you have been told that you are unlikely to give birth to a child or that it would be unwise for you to do so, you may like to consider the possibility of adoption or fostering. But don't do this too hastily. While it can be an excellent thing to do – both for the sake of the parents and of a child who might otherwise spend his or her life in care – it is something to be carefully thought about and not entered into as some sort of knee-jerk reaction to a miscarriage.

- If the above does not apply, most doctors say that it is all right to try for another baby after you have had two normal periods. But, while it is all right to do so, whether you are ready or not is entirely up to you. We are all different and we react in different ways so only you will know when the time is right to try to become pregnant again.

- Having been through the awful experience of a miscarriage (or more than one), it is only natural to feel afraid of what might happen during a future pregnancy. But statistics show that even those who have been unfortunate enough to suffer three miscarriages still have a more than 50 per cent chance of a successful pregnancy and labour in the future.

  We have seen that many doctors do not treat miscarriage as a real problem until the woman has suffered three. If you don't want to wait and see if this happens to you, you could arrange to have a consultation with a specialist – ask either your doctor or the local branch of the Miscarriage Association for the name of such a specialist.

- Before even attempting to become pregnant again, contact Foresight so that you and your partner can do everything possible to prepare yourselves for a healthy pregnancy and the birth of a healthy child. At the same time, use your own common-sense when it comes to nutrition, exercise, relaxation, etc.

- It has been shown that outside emotional support at such a time can prove to be positively beneficial, so consult your midwife or a complementary therapist to be helped in this way.

- If you are using the pill as your means of contraception, try to find an alternative method for about six months prior to trying to become pregnant again.

4. WHEN PREGNANT

- Avoid all alcohol if possible – particularly spirits and red wine.
- Give up smoking if you have not already done so. Apart from the long-term damage it can do to both you and the baby, smoking can more than double the chance of having a miscarriage.
- Avoid any form of heavy lifting and refrain from dragging heavy objects from place to place.
- Make sure that you have plenty of rest, especially when the stage at which you had the miscarriage approaches. You cannot totally avoid the stress that will arise but try to practise a deep relaxation technique.
- Obtain expert advice on diet, nutrition, vitamin and mineral needs, etc. Not only will it be better for your health – and the baby's – but the knowledge that you are taking positive control of the situation will help to boost your confidence.
- Follow your own instincts when it comes to making plans for the baby and how detailed these plans should be. If past experience has made you wary of planning, buying or decorating, leave it until later. However, should you feel able to prepare in this practical way for the baby, go ahead and do it. It is important to act in a way which is comfortable for you and not the way in which someone else thinks you should act.
- Take time every day to commune with your unborn child by sitting or lying quietly – perhaps with some gentle music in the background. Spend this time talking to the baby – either aloud or inside your head – reassuring him or her of your love, explaining how wanted he or she is and generally talking about the wonderful future you are going to have together. It has been proved time and again that doing this keeps the baby calm and contented in the womb and also makes for a more relaxed infant after birth.

- Make use of any of the complementary therapies described in the previous chapter, being sure that you tell the therapist that you are pregnant when you first go to see them, even if nothing is visible as yet. This will naturally make a difference to any remedies you might be given or to the type of exercise or massage you will receive.

- Enjoy your pregnancy. Just because something went wrong before does not mean that the same thing will happen again. Think how many times you fell over as a child – yet you don't spend your adult life in dread in case you fall again. Try not to spoil what can be a beautiful time in your life by being preoccupied with the past – spend that time instead feeling happy and fulfilled and anticipating the joy that is to be yours when your baby is born.

CONCLUSION

Although a miscarriage is a sad and distressing occurrence, it is a fact that, unless there is some deep underlying physical problem, most women who suffer a miscarriage go on to give birth to one or more healthy children. It is important to keep this in mind as you look towards your future and the family you hope to have.

Further Reading

Allen, M and Marks, S, *Miscarriage, Sharing from the Heart*, Wiley, Chichester, 1993

Hill, S, *Family*, Michael Joseph, London, 1989

Ilse, S and Hammer Burns, L, *Empty Arms*, Wintergreen, USA, 1990

Markham, U, *The Element Guide: Bereavement*, Element Books, Shaftesbury, 1996

Markham, U, *Elements of Visualization*, Element Books, Shaftesbury, 1993

Markham, U, *Women and Guilt*, Piatkus Books, London, 1995

Pickard, B, *Eating Well for a Healthy Pregnancy*, Sheldon Press, London, 1984

CASSETTES

Ursula Markham's self-hypnosis cassettes and courses are available from:

The Hypnothink Foundation
PO Box 66
Gloucester
GL2 9YG
United Kingdom

Useful Addresses

United Kingdom

The resources of all these organizations are greatly stretched and each would be grateful for a stamped, self-addressed envelope when you contact them.

The Miscarriage Association
Clayton Hospital
Northgate
Wakefield, West Yorkshire
WF1 3JS

Foresight (Pre-Conceptual Care)
28 The Paddock
Godalming, Surrey
GU7 1XD

SANDS (Stillbirth and Neonatal Death Society)
28 Portland Place
London
W1N 3DE

CRUSE (support for the bereaved)
Cruse House
126 Sheen Road
Richmond, Surrey
TW9 1UR

British Association for Counselling
1 Regent Place
Rugby, Warwickshire
CV21 2PJ

Compassionate Friends
53 North Street
Bristol
BS3 1EN

Foundation for Black Bereaved Families
11 Kingston Square
Salters Hill, London
SE19 1DZ

Jewish Bereavement Counselling Service

126 Albert Street
London
NW1 1NF

United States of America

Compassionate Friends
PO Box 3696
Oak Brook
Illinois 60522–3696

55 Commonwealth Avenue
Kenmore Square
Boston
MA 02215

386 Stanley Street
Fall River
MA 02720

PO Box 12004
Hartford
CT 06112

PO Box 832
Keene
NH 03431

2013 Elm Street
Manchester
NH 03404

2 Magee Street
Providence
RI 02906

PO Box 1259
New York
NY 10159

PO Box 9814
Washington
DC 20016

Pregnancy and Infant Loss
   Center
1421E Wayzata Boulevard,
   Suite 30
Wayzata
MN 55391-1939

Foresight U.S.
Woodlands Health
   Center
5724 Clymer Road
Quakertown
PA 18591

Australia

Compassionate Friends
9 Carlisle Avenue
Morphettville 5043
Adelaide

79 Stirling Street
Perth
WA 6000

PO Box 218
Springwood
Queensland 4127

Bereaved Parents' Support
   Centre
Lower Parish Hall
300 Camberwell Road
Camberwell 3124
Melbourne

Foresight Australia
124 Louisa Road
Birch Grove 2041
New South Wales

Complementary Therapists

For details of a therapist in your area, contact the offices listed.

HYPNOTHERAPY

United Kingdom

The Hypnotherapy Register
The Hypnothink Foundation
PO Box 66
Gloucester
GL2 9YG

The National Council for
    Hypnotherapy
Hazelwood
Broadmead, Sway
Lymington, Hants
SO41 6DH

United States of America

American Association of
    Professional
    Hypnotherapists
PO Box 29
Boones Mill
VA 24065

Australia

Australian School for Clinical
    and Experimental Hypnosis
Royal Melbourne Hospital
Royal Parade
Parkville
Victoria

AROMATHERAPY

United Kingdom

Shirley Price Aromatherapy
Essentia House
Upper Bond Street
Hinckley, Leicestershire
LE10 1RS

United States of America

Margot Latimer
    Aromatherapy
PO Box 65
Pineville
PA 18946

Australia

Australian School of
	Awareness
PO Box 187
Montrose 3765

HOMEOPATHY

United Kingdom

British Homeopathic
	Association
27A Devonshire Street
London
W1N 1RJ

United States of America

National Center for
	Homeopathy
801 North Fairfax Street, Suite
	306
Alexandria
VA 22314

Australia

Australian Federation of
	Homeopaths
PO Box 806
Spit Junction
New South Wales 2088

ALEXANDER TECHNIQUE

United Kingdom

Society of Teachers of the
	Alexander Technique

266 Fulham Road
London
SW10 9EL

United States of America

NASTAT
3010 Hennepin Avenue South,
	Suite 10
Minneapolis
MN 55408

Australia

AUSTAT
PO Box 716
Darlinghurst
New South Wales 2010

BACH FLOWER REMEDIES

United Kingdom

The Dr Edward Bach Centre
Mount Vernon
Sotwell, Wallingford
Oxfordshire
OX10 0PZ

ACUPUNCTURE

United Kingdom

College of Oriental Medicine
Prospect House
2 Grove Lane
Retford, Notts
DN22 6NA

United States of America

National Acupuncture and
  Oriental Medicine Alliance
1833 North 105th Street
Seattle
WA 98133

Australia

Australian Acupuncture
  Ethics and Standards
Organization
PO Box 84
Merrylands
New South Wales 2160

HERBAL MEDICINE
(WESTERN)

United Kingdom

National Institute of Medical
  Herbalists
56 Longbrook Street
Exeter EX4 6AH

United States of America

National College of
  Phytotherapy
10401 Montgomery Park Way
  NE
Albuquerque
NM 87111

Austrlia

National Herbalists'
  Association of Australia

Suite 14, 247 Kingsgrove Road
Kingsgrove
New South Wales 2208

HERBAL MEDICINE
(CHINESE)

United Kingdom

College of Oriental Medicine
Prospect House
2 Grove Lane
Retford, Notts
DN22 6NA

United States of America

National Acupuncture and
  Oriental Medicine Alliance
1833N 105th Street
Seattle
WA 98133

NUTRITIONAL THERAPY

United Kingdom

Society for the Promotion of
  Nutritional Therapy
PO Box 47
Heathfield, East Sussex
TN21 8ZK

United States of America

Kushi Institute
17 Station Street
Brookline Village
MA 02147

Index